CHANGE IS POSSIBLE

CHANGE IS POSSIBLE

Reflections on the History of Global Health

William H. Foege

Paul Elish

Alison T. Hoover

Madison Gabriella Lee

Deborah Chen Tseng

Kiera Chan

JOHNS HOPKINS UNIVERSITY PRESS | *Baltimore*

© 2024 Johns Hopkins University Press
All rights reserved. Published 2024
Printed in the United States of America on acid-free paper
9 8 7 6 5 4 3 2 1

Johns Hopkins University Press
2715 North Charles Street
Baltimore, Maryland 21218
www.press.jhu.edu

Library of Congress Cataloging-in-Publication Data is available.

A catalog record for this book is available from the British Library.

ISBN 978-1-4214-5042-1 (paperback)
ISBN 978-1-4214-5043-8 (ebook)

Special discounts are available for bulk purchases of this book. For more information, please contact Special Sales at specialsales@jh.edu.

To Joanne Amposta Williams, Tom Paulson, and Anne Mather

CONTENTS

Change Is Possible: Reflections on the History of Global Health

BILL FOEGE WITH TOM PAULSON

This book is both a chronicle of major influencers of global health and a personal history. I was privileged to have been in the field long enough to have witnessed many, if not most, of the transformative events that have shaped current global health activities—some for the better, others arguably for the worse.

As a teenager, temporarily confined to a single position in a body cast for months due to a hip disorder, I read about Albert Schweitzer and was inspired to try to follow his path by doing medical work in Africa. This was the medical missionary phase that preceded modern global health. I learned the hard way that such "charitable" approaches to medicine, though often helpful in terms of providing direct care, can have negative impacts unforeseen by even the most well-intentioned.

Growing up in rural eastern Washington State, I spent several summers fighting wildland fires. Fire often serves as a metaphor for infectious disease, and firefighting can just as well serve as a metaphor for battling the spread of disease. Repeatedly, this metaphor became reality during the smallpox-eradication campaign. When faced with a shortage of vaccines during an outbreak, my colleagues and I decided to use a strategy employed by forest firefighters—encircling the blaze with a fuel-free ring so the fire can't spread for lack of fuel. The approach was not new. It had been advocated by an 1898 Royal Commission that studied a century of experience with smallpox. At that time, compulsory vaccination laws were common; however, a strong antivaccination movement in Leicester resulted in a program that emphasized quarantine of cases and vaccination of those who had contact with cases. In the smallpox campaign, we were forced to try it for lack of vaccine. And it worked.

Thus was born an approach that removed the first half of the World Health Organization's strategy, namely, mass vaccination. WHO had always intended to concentrate on every outbreak of smallpox, but only after an expensive campaign of mass vaccination. This so-called ring vaccination strategy hastened the eradication of smallpox. While *ring vaccination* is often used to describe the strategy, in fact "surveillance/containment" had three elements: quarantine of case-patients, vaccination of those at highest risk of contact with cases, and an active search for new cases.

In this book, you will discover other surprising twists and turns that built the foundation upon which global health stands. You will learn that the greatest disaster for global health improvement was colonialism, and surprisingly, that the greatest asset for global health improvement may well have been military medicine. You may disagree but hear us out. You may also be surprised to learn that Johns Hopkins was not the first academic program in this country providing diplomas for global health.

I love history but cannot claim to be a historian. Winston Churchill said, "History will be kind to me, for I intend to write it." To reduce the risk of burdening this book with too many of my personal biases, I enlisted five public health students at Emory University to research and write up different categories and phases of global health: Paul Elish, Alison T. Hoover, Madison Gabriella Lee, Deborah Chen Tseng, and Kiera Chan. Two writer-editors I have known for decades, Anne Mather and Tom Paulson, assisted in cleaning up our copy and improving the narrative. My wife, Paula, gave important advice on making chapters readable. This project could not have been done without all of them. Although all of us had the chance to opine on every chapter, we list the lead author. This is simple courtesy, but it also reminds me of an early mentor who told me the first lesson of management is to learn how to delegate blame!

Dean Jim Curran of the Rollins School of Public Health supported the students with financial stipends. Joanne Amposta Williams provided the support structure for the students as they organized their contributions. She also provided for our biweekly Zoom sessions for us all to discuss and comment on research findings—a balm during the forced isolation of COVID-19. Indeed, we met face to face only once, in January 2020, at Emory University, but conducted biweekly sessions for a year by Zoom. After each session, I was impressed by what I had learned from the students' research.

And it was the students who suggested the name for this book. I was delighted, as "Change Is Possible" was the motto for the Marguerite Casey Foundation work on behalf of young people especially burdened by poverty, educational challenges, and adverse social determinants of health and well-being. For years, I was on the board of this important endeavor.

Why spend time on history? It is not to avoid mistakes. We will continue to make mistakes no matter how much history we read. The purpose of reading history is to become absolutely convinced that this is a cause-and-effect world, not a world of magic. We won't understand all of the causes, but we will become convinced that every action we take today will have consequences that go on forever. This should make us more aware that we awake each morning making history for the future.

And we will see that everything—from coronavirus and monkeypox actions today, to the most earnest endeavors of well-motivated global health workers throughout history—has aspects of triumph and tragedy. It is an exciting attempt to understand what actually worked and what made life harder—to make each of us cognizant of the future we are constructing for others. If we could be true to our vision of causes and effects, we would have to list countless people who influenced each author and helped to uncover source material. Instead, we are reduced to the poor substitute of thanking everyone.

There will continue to be arguments on the definition of global health. Being of simplistic thinking, I simply abbreviate it to any activity that promotes "global health equity." It is not possible to improve the meaning by removing any one of the 3 words, but it is not made clearer by the addition of 200 words.

CHANGE IS POSSIBLE

CHAPTER 1

The Triumph and Tragedy of Global Health

BILL FOEGE

There was no reason, in the 1940s, to think that global health might be a future interest. My first 10 years were spent in rural Iowa, attending a one-room school with only two classmates for the first five years. On Pearl Harbor Day, with parents visiting sick church members and a friend staying with me and four siblings, we heard the news on the radio, but we didn't even know where Pearl Harbor was. When we moved to northeast Washington State, to a town of 1,500 people, it seemed an enormous change, as our Iowa town had had only 100 people, but we were still relatively isolated.

At age 15, I was put in a body cast, as I mentioned in the preface, unable to turn over, get up, or even move for some months. So, I became a reader in a town lacking television. Reading *Out of My Life and Thought* by Albert Schweitzer was a turning point. I could not appreciate what it meant for someone to be so brilliant that he had earned three doctoral degrees before age 30. If that was not enough, he was also an accomplished organist, the world's authority on both Bach and organ building. He had a brilliant career ahead of him. Instead, he went to medical school for a fourth degree, in medicine, and spent over half a century in what is now Gabon, to provide healthcare for people who had no idea how different their experience was compared to others in Africa.

For the next 70 years, the idea of global health equity influenced my decisions. Over those 70 years, global health eliminated some problems. It saved millions of children from an early death, many from blindness, and provided hope, as this book will show.

And then, in 2020, we had a new experience, predicted for decades, but somehow worse than expected. It was the most frightening new virus in a century: efficient at finding new victims, ruthless in cutting off oxygen, leaving people gasping for breath, and killing in numbers that left response systems devastated. But then, it was made even worse by a response in the United States that simply ignored the lessons painfully learned since the germ theory was first understood.

Stephen Hawking said the history of science was the gradual realization that things do not happen in arbitrary ways. But President Donald Trump said COVID-19 would disappear, as if by magic. A basic requirement in public health is to know the truth. But the daily White House press briefings gave "alternative truths."

History taught public health workers that a national health threat required a coordinated national response, which would allow states, counties, cities, territories, and tribes to modify plans based on local conditions. Paraphrasing, the White House said to the states, "You are on your own. Figure out a plan and compete with each other to obtain resources and supplies."

History also taught that the best decisions are based on the best science, while the best results are based on the best management. The White House gagged the Centers for Disease Control and Prevention (CDC) and actually altered the CDC website to cause confusion. This compromised both scientific decisions and strong management.

Basic public health understands globalization, where everything affects everything. Yet the White House decided to leave the World Health Organization in the midst of a pandemic. When we thought nature could not hurt us more, we found that human incompetence could combine with nature to cause even greater pain.

And so, we added yet another lesson to what history has taught us, namely, lessons are meaningless if ignored. As Mark Twain said, the person who doesn't read has no advantage over the person who can't read. The country that ignores public health lessons is no better off than a country living before the germ theory was understood.

In the midst of this tragedy, a vaccine was quickly developed. Not only was it good, it was spectacular. And over time it became clear that this dangerous virus was easily outsmarted by science. It was helpless in the face of messenger RNA vaccines, viral vector vaccines, and protein vaccines. So, it then relied on evolution, to mutate in an attempt to outmaneuver the vaccine.

How could the same political group that thwarted a reasonable public health response have supported this breakthrough in science and technology? The reason may be as simple as the comfort people feel in making public health pronouncements. It is easy for the president to say the problem will disappear as if by magic, or for Dr. Scott W. Atlas to say herd immunity is the answer. But very few people believe they can make a vaccine. So, the same politicians that blocked public health measures were able to give money to the National Institutes of Health and corporations to produce a vaccine, and then stay out of their way.

While politics weakened public health in combating the coronavirus, another new problem, monkeypox, soon surfaced. The monkeypox virus had similarities to smallpox, producing a clinical picture that mimicked modified smallpox, but it spread more slowly. A half century of experience in Africa showed that transmission in humans would often cease after two or three generations of the disease.

However, monkeypox virus also could evolve and spread more rapidly in the environment of gay sex. A response of hyperactive surveillance and careful containment practices, as practiced in India with smallpox, would have been an appropriate response. But at the time of writing this, such an effort has lagged.

How did we get to this point of combining chaos and scientific excellence? We have been eyewitnesses to triumph and tragedy with coronavirus. But it is no exception: triumph and tragedy have been factors in every step of the global health journey.

Global health is an amalgamation of ingredients and historical developments over the centuries. This book roughly follows the sequence of actual events: the colonial expansion, military health involvement, church medical missions, academic global health studies, bilateral health programs, multilateral health plans, nongovernmental projects, corporation support, and finally new resources from philanthropy. But we start with a chapter on politics and global health, potentially the most powerful combination for providing global health equity in the future.

Certainty is the Achilles heel of science, according to Richard Feynman, so we approach this with great humility. Nonetheless, we can say with a high degree of certainty that we will see another pandemic, perhaps greater than that of COVID-19. The world has experienced, on average, a new infectious disease problem each year for decades: Lassa fever, hemorrhagic fevers of various kinds, Ebola in 1976 and again in 2014, toxic shock syndrome, HIV, Zika, SARS, MERS, and coronavirus to name some recent ones.

It will continue to happen. So, we look back in order to plan forward.

Each chapter in this book was researched, and an original draft written, by the graduate public health students mentioned in the preface, who attended the Rollins School of Public Health, Emory University. They are listed as primary authors for the sections they researched and drafted. Modifications followed, and an attempt was made to identify some triumphs and tragedies, in a concluding paragraph for each chapter. Much attention is devoted to the roles of colonialism and militaries: the authors regard colonialism as having had the greatest negative impact on global health, while military medicine, surprisingly, may have had the greatest positive impact.

To meld the various voices, Tom Paulson and Anne Mather provided overarching harmony to make this a choir rather than individual vocalists. We then circled back to comment on the attempts to extract the world from the COVID-19 nightmare and to prepare for the future. It is an exciting journey of courage, suffering, mistakes of all kinds, and foibles, all combining to better understand the health of the world today.

CHAPTER 2

Politics and Global Health

BILL FOEGE

When we started our medical careers in the 1950s, we were very naïve. We assumed that both medicine and public health could be pure pursuits, not tainted by political involvement. Medical schools still had the quaint belief that medical decisions for an individual were made by the patient and the doctor; they believed that approach would continue. The concept of rules imposed by government and insurance companies to limit such decisions was on the horizon, feared but not in clear focus. The American Medical Association bombarded us students with messages to beware of socialized medicine and to look over our shoulder to avoid having the concept gain ground.

It took time to realize that true socialized medicine involves the government actually owning hospitals and clinics, as in the United Kingdom. Those promoting what was called socialized medicine in the United States were actually trying to expand funding for specific groups.

Never did we get messages to look over the other shoulder to watch for restrictions on medical practice imposed by capitalism. The marketplace was the gold standard; there was no inkling that it would be a greater threat to health than socialism. Even with a thousand deaths a day, year after year, due to tobacco, free enterprise continued to determine the approach to, and the thinking of, healthcare professionals.

Our thinking about medical practice spilled over to public health. We thought our decisions could be pure, accepted, and financed. We assumed that good scientific proposals would be embraced by politicians and adequately financed.

We missed the fact that public health and politics are so intertwined that much of public health is already funded by government; hence, the two cannot be separated. In reality, public health is already close to a single-payer system. There are public health activities supported by some corporations, churches, or academic institutions; however, in general, government supports most public health activities. Therefore, the power of an appropriation system means politicians will cast the final vote regarding public health programs. Medical ethics has traditionally focused closely on decisions affecting the beginning and end of life. However, the real battleground for medical ethics is found in budget decisions. They describe our priorities; our tradeoffs; our understanding of the ingredients of life quality, unnecessary suffering, and premature mortality. Public health workers, therefore, need to understand the appropriation system and how to provide politicians with the information they need to make good decisions.

Prevention, good health, and community approaches inspire great lip service. Yet repeatedly we find that individuals, families, communities, nations, and indeed the world value health most when they lose it. Just as we learn about geology the day after an earthquake, we learn about public health when faced with an emergency.

A study by the Carter Center in 1985 found that two of every three deaths in the United States were premature, given the knowledge already available. We simply were not funding prevention and public health to realize those outcomes. Likewise, cancer research concentrated on funding basic research, despite the fact that one-third of all cancers were already preventable (with tobacco being the chief villain) and one-third were treatable. The funding of prevention programs was not valued as highly as basic research, so premature deaths and unnecessary suffering resulted.

Over the years it became evident that political will was an essential ingredient in improving the health of the public. The work of Senator

J. Lister Hill, in 1955, changed forever the ability of this country to use the power of vaccines for all children in the country. Through the years, other political heroes, who became invested in public health and helped to secure appropriations, have emerged.

In 1993, Michael McGinnis and I published a paper on the real causes of death in this country.[1] Death certificates list the proximal causes, such as heart attacks, strokes, and cancer. But looking behind those numbers, one realizes that 40% of all deaths were actually due to tobacco, diet, and alcohol. Medical practitioners see the impact late in the progression of disease. They are not reimbursed for time spent on prevention and, therefore, it is often neglected. Working to prevent the impact of these conditions requires public health approaches, political support, and changes in reimbursement for those working in clinics and hospitals. Indeed, legislators increasing tobacco taxes actually had more impact than those treating tobacco-related conditions. And lawyers had an impact on politicians that was not enjoyed by public health practitioners.

Recent decades have made it increasingly clear that we need additional attention to the causes behind the causes. Social determinants such as poverty, unemployment, gender bias, lack of educational opportunities, and racism all impact health. Medicine must be involved, especially in reducing poverty and racism, but politicians hold the greatest power in addressing these social conditions.

Evolution of My Thinking

At a time before I fully appreciated the need for political involvement in public health, I expressed anger at a congressional decision that would worsen public health. My deputy director at the CDC, Bill Watson, said it was actually my fault. He said if I had anticipated the information that the politicians needed before making their decision, they would probably have arrived at a different conclusion. This, of course, was at a time when facts still mattered.

Bill's comment led me to try to anticipate and inform politicians. My efforts were partially successful. But this took an incredible amount of work because of congressional turnover and because politicians' levels of interest in public health did not always match ours. This led to the third step in my thinking about politics and public health: actual participation. I now remind students of public health that some of them should consider politics. It would be a much more efficient system if public health–trained people were in congressional and government positions.

There have been notable examples of this approach. One is Dr. Gro Brundtland, who was trained in medicine and public health and later became prime minister of Norway. That background served her well when she chaired a global report on the environment and later became the director-general of the World Health Organization (WHO).

President Carter and Global Health

But sometimes a politician does become interested in public health. President Jimmy Carter is the prime example. Following his years in the White House, he established the Carter Center in Atlanta. His early concerns involved having a place for conflict resolution. His Camp David experience in bringing peace between Egypt and Israel had fired his imagination about what might be done—and it provided experience in how to do it. He also foresaw that election monitoring would be a valuable asset to provide countries seeking a road to democracy. His political ties around the world and his easy access to country leaders made such efforts logical and doable.

In the first conversation we had in his exploration of my interest in becoming executive director of the Carter Center, I found myself surprised and flattered. But I pointed out my lack of experience in those areas, and also the fact that my life and passion had revolved around global health. At that time, so few people were going into that field that it seemed inappropriate to abandon it. (Thankfully, the past 30 years have seen an unprecedented interest in global health, and student applications in the field have soared.)

This was before I understood President Carter to be a polymath, a person interested in everything. He seemed to accept my explanation, but then returned some days later with the question, "Would it change your mind if I also became interested in global health?"

What an unbelievable opportunity. What might happen to the field if he became involved? I took him at his word, accepted his offer, and found myself in an arena that was novel, scary, and exciting.

At the time, I was heading a task force formed by WHO, UNICEF, the United Nations Development Programme, the World Bank, and the Rockefeller Foundation. The task force was called the Task Force for Child Survival. It is now the Task Force for Global Health. It has expanded its mission from childhood immunization to global health in general and especially the promotion of work on neglected diseases. The Carter Center was new and had extra space. So, the Task Force rented space in the Carter Center building, and I could be involved in both projects simultaneously, from a single office.

Closing the Gap Addresses Domestic Needs

The first Carter Center health project concerned domestic health. President Carter and Assistant Secretary for Health Dr. Ed Brandt co-chaired a meeting on the subject November 26–28, 1984.

If we needed any proof that involving a politician in public health could be beneficial, that meeting made the case. The basic question it aimed to answer was, "If we had no additional research findings, what could happen to morbidity and mortality if we simply implemented what we know?"

Public health professionals were eager to participate, and the breadth of the preparatory papers was staggering in terms of completeness and professionalism. Background papers were developed on alcohol dependence and abuse, arthritis and musculoskeletal diseases, cancer, cardiovascular disease, dental disease, depression, diabetes, digestive diseases, drug dependency, infectious and parasitic diseases, respiratory diseases, socioeconomic status and health, unintended pregnancy and infant mortality, unintentional injuries, and intended violence. President Carter and Brandt both contributed articles to the resulting publication.

The meeting was reported in the *Journal of the American Medical Association*:[2]

> A NATIONAL consultation on health policy . . . was cochaired by former President Jimmy Carter and Edward N. Brandt, Jr, MD, Assistant Secretary for Health. Contributions appear in this issue from President Carter . . . and Dr Brandt. . . . Rather than seek technologic breakthroughs, the project seeks to focus national health policy on the "gap" represented by health problems that are unnecessary in light of knowledge that already is at hand. Consultants from various medical specialties conducted extensive investigations of the burden.

The meeting result was clear and somewhat surprising. Two of every three deaths in the United States were premature, given our state of knowledge. This is a staggering, preventable tragedy. But it is not only deaths; much of the burden of illness in this country was unnecessary, given our skills and knowledge. The study also indicated what could be done to improve delivery and research.

President and Mrs. Carter were so impressed with the meeting and the findings that they jointly wrote a book giving their personal experiences and beliefs to make this information available to the public.[3]

Closing the Gap Globally

A second ambitious project of the Carter Center attempted a similar evaluation of the global health and disease situation. From April 27 to May 1, 1986, at a meeting titled "Risks Old and New: A Global Consultation on Health," ministers of health and others working in global health reviewed old problems and new opportunities. Again, the spirited discussion and sharing of experiences proved the value of President Carter's engaging in public health.

One searing memory of that meeting was a reception my wife, Paula, and I had at our house for participants. The minister of health from Kyiv had just learned of the nuclear disaster at Chernobyl. The parameters of the problem were still unknown, but he was in a state of high anxiety because he had been told not to return home. The reason given was that the Soviet Union was uncertain of the extent of the problem and did not want to frighten the world by suddenly recalling a top health official.

The consultations were important in selecting the problems for Carter Center focus. President Carter had no interest in competing in areas where other groups had programs. He was especially attracted to problems of the poor and often forgotten populations.

Neglected Diseases

Soon, much of the Carter Center activity involved neglected diseases. Guinea worm eradication became an obsession. Dr. Don Hopkins led the effort to eradicate this blight. Dracunculiasis is caused by a parasite, *Dracunculus medinensis*, which infects humans when they ingest a water flea containing a larval form of the parasite. Once ingested, it develops in the lymph system of humans, with the female reaching a length of two to three feet. After about 12 months, the worm seeks to release thousands of eggs. The worm accomplishes this when its distal end surfaces on a person's skin, usually in the foot or ankle. The worm breaks through the skin when a person steps into water, at which point it discharges its eggs. The eggs are consumed by water fleas and changed into a new larval form capable of reinfecting humans.

The lesion on the ankle may be painful and become infected. The worm is often removed slowly over a period of days or weeks. Often, it is pulled out an inch or two, wrapped around a matchstick, and bandaged until the next day. Those suffering are often unable to work in the fields or to attend school. A single person may have a dozen painful worms emerging, not all confined to the lower leg. Worms can exit any place and are so unsightly that people often want to hide from public view. In Nigeria, dracunculiasis was found to be the single most important reason for missing school.

President Carter went directly to the head of state, President Ibrahim Babangida, to seek support for the program. Ministries of health were often unaware of the problem since it was not seen in cities. The extent of the disease was demonstrated in Nigeria when an active prevalence search was done. Nigeria typically reported a few thousand cases a year. Yet, at a single point in time, searchers found almost 700,000 active cases. The president of Nigeria was so impressed that he pledged $1 million of Nigerian resources to counter this problem.

This turned out to be the pattern for many programs. President Carter would go directly to the head of state to discuss dracunculiasis, schistosomiasis, onchocerciasis, trachoma, lymphatic filariasis, sanitation systems, vaccination programs, polio eradication, and other health problems.

Regardless of their experiences in tropical countries, no medical members of the Carter Center, upon visiting another country, could expect to get an appointment with anyone above the position of minister of health. Even the minister of finance, a potent force in helping or hindering health activities, would not agree to meetings. But for President Carter, the head of state would often call a meeting that included the cabinet, and proposals were discussed with all of its members. If the head of state became convinced, participation was easy.

Several meetings with flight lieutenant Jerry Rawlings, president of Ghana, led to Rawlings personally touring the country and demonstrating how to interrupt the Guinea worm cycle, even to the point of filtering water from a pond and then drinking the water to demonstrate its safety. This caused great concern when Carter Center staff learned of this practice, since the filtering removed the water flea but not bacteria and viruses, which could cause other problems.

Because of President Carter's access to heads of state—and the unrelenting work of Dr. Hopkins—the annual burden of Guinea worm was reduced from millions of cases a year to thousands, then hundreds, and now a handful a year. Eradication appears imminent.

A similar story was repeated for onchocerciasis (river blindness), as outlined in another chapter. Merck started the process, but the marketing involved President Carter, again with visits to heads of state.

Soon President Carter was promoting an attack on trachoma. It is a significant cause of blindness in Africa and has been reduced with the help of Pfizer, which donated an antibiotic to treat the infection, plus the training of health workers to perform surgical approaches to the disease. In addition, training in hygiene to prevent spread of the organism became an integral part of the program.

Many of these diseases had not afflicted the United States. However, we did have well- documented problems with hookworm, malaria, yellow fever, and cholera. And even trachoma has caused blindness in this country until recently, especially in Native American populations. The greatest athlete of the 20th century, Jim Thorpe, had eye surgery for trachoma in 1911, the year before his spectacular performance in the 1912 Olympic Games. One of the early smallpox-eradication workers, Dr. Stan Foster, began his public health career working on trachoma with Native American tribes in 1962.

President Carter's role in the beginning of the lymphatic filariasis program has been mentioned previously. Add to that a program to expand the use of outhouses; promotions to reduce the toll of vaccine-preventable diseases, especially polio; HIV prevention; and numerous other projects. The breadth of these programs demonstrates the value of a concerned politician assisting in improvements in global health.

Inspiring Other Leaders

President Carter also inspired other political leaders to become interested in health as a general topic, not simply an interest in one or two programs. General Amadou Toumani Touré, in Mali, began working with Guinea worm disease at the urging of Carter, but he continued to support health programs when he was president of Mali. General Yakubu Gowan of Nigeria became an active participant in the Guinea worm eradication program and later became very active in programs against AIDS and malaria. President Yoweri Museveni of Uganda became involved in AIDS as well as child survival programs. Carter's influence extended throughout the African region, in efforts to improve health conditions.

The death of Gary Strieker in July 2022 provides a glimpse of President Carter's activities. The periodic publication for Guinea worm eradication[4] noted:

We share with heavy hearts the news that Gary Strieker died this month. Among his many accomplishments, Gary worked nearly twenty years for CNN, including as CNN's bureau chief in Nairobi. It was in the latter role that he accompanied former U.S. President Jimmy Carter, at Carter's invitation, from Nairobi to Khartoum, Sudan in March 1995 to document and broadcast the famous "Guinea Worm Cease-Fire" agreement between the warring sides in Sudan's long civil war. As a prolific film producer and director, he accompanied President and Mrs. Carter on an epic four country tour initiated by then-Carter Center Board of Directors Chair John Moores to visit Carter Center-assisted health projects in Ghana, Sudan/southern Sudan, Ethiopia, and Nigeria in 2007. The tour focused on Guinea worm eradication in all four countries, as well as on onchocerciasis, lymphatic filariasis, and schistosomiasis in Nigeria; onchocerciasis and malaria bed net distribution in Ethiopia; and trachoma in Ghana. In 2010 he produced the award-winning feature film about Guinea worm eradication, "Foul Water/Fiery Serpent."[5]

The article on Strieker highlights multiple programs in multiple countries.

Malnutrition

One feature of disease in Africa that is obvious but not often mentioned is the burden of multiple and simultaneous health insults. In the mid-20th century, clinicians in Africa often saw a child with a presenting complaint of measles. But at the same time, that child might have malaria parasites in the blood, Guinea worms and filaria in the lymph system, schistosomes in the bladder, hookworms and roundworms in the intestine—plus malnutrition. Some would see it as gross malpractice to deal only with a single disease. But the truth is that the removal of any one of these problems could improve health and survival. Every health improvement was always inadequate, nonetheless a positive step, a shining light on a dark background of unmet needs.

One of the most interesting programs involved the attempt to improve nutrition in Africa. Many of the deaths attributed to measles, malaria, diarrhea, and pneumonia were directly due to malnutrition.

Norman Borlaug, 1970 Nobel laureate for his work in improving wheat production in India and Pakistan, became a consultant to the Carter Center to see what would be required to improve agriculture in Africa. In 1962, Ryōichi Sasakawa had started the Nippon Foundation in Japan. Sasakawa had been suspected of being a war criminal but was eventually set free and developed motorboat racing in Japan. The Nippon Foundation was originally set up to provide profits from motorboat racing to improve Japan's ship building, provide programs for young people, and other domestic projects. The Ethiopian famine in the mid-1980s led Sasakawa to develop agricultural education programs in Africa. At that time, Sasakawa reached out to Norman Borlaug, suggesting an expansion of the Carter Center's agricultural program. Borlaug attempted to beg off, citing his age. But Sasakawa discounted that explanation, pointing out that *he* was older than Borlaug. The combination of Carter, Borlaug, and Sasakawa turned out to be inspired.

Programs were started in multiple countries. Without fail, the projects taught farmers how to space seeds, use the correct amount of fertilizer, protect crops at harvest time, and provide storage of harvested grains to reduce loss to rodents. In every case, productivity increased by 200% to 400%. But it was difficult to change governmental approaches to capitalize on these techniques. It requires government support to have seed and fertilizer available at the right time. It requires government subsidies to allow farmers to buy seed and fertilizer. It requires government support to provide local and regional storage to avoid a drop in prices at harvest and major increases in prices before the next harvest. It requires government support to provide improved roads to make use of trucking or other transport. To date, most African governments have found it difficult to take these reasonable actions for future prosperity.

One significant aspect of the agricultural program was the introduction of high-protein maize to Africa. Maize lacks two essential amino acids, lysine and tryptophan. Since humans cannot make these amino acids, their presence in the diet is essential. In maize-eating societies, children are often breastfed until the next child is born. At that point, they are weaned on a gruel of maize and can develop protein malnutrition even if adequate maize is available. These children are then at higher risk of death if they acquire measles, other infectious diseases, or diarrhea.

Dr. Cicely Williams described this condition, in 1935, while she was working in what was then called the Gold Coast. She suggested that it was due to a diet deficient in protein and used the word *kwashiorkor*, a name from the Ga language in Ghana, referring to the disease an infant gets when a new sibling is born.

Norman Borlaug and I were with President Carter during a visit to see President Jerry Rawlings to discuss Guinea worm. Borlaug related to me the story of Quality Protein Maize (QPM), developed by Surinder Vasal and Evangelina Villegas at the International Maize and Wheat Improvement Center in Mexico. This was the research station where Borlaug had improved wheat strains years earlier. Borlaug said QPM could change malnutrition rates in a place like Ghana if it were accepted by farmers. He then related the many steps that had been taken to make the strain acceptable. It had to have the same color and firmness of maize already in use. It had to be resistant to fungus and shown to grow in African soil. He felt that all of these measures had now been achieved, but he was concerned it would take many years for farmers to accept it.

Relating the story to President Carter resulted in his immediate interest. He invited us to have dinner with President Rawlings. President Carter right away related the story about QPM. He then asked Borlaug to describe QPM's agricultural implications and me to describe its nutritional benefits. I told President Rawlings that I had three messages. First, the problem had been described from Ghana in 1935 by Dr. Cicely Williams, using the Ghanaian word *kwashiorkor*. Second, it would be fitting for the solution to emanate from Ghana. Third, it would be wonderful to have that happen in the lifetime of Cicely Williams.

President Rawlings looked surprised and asked, "Is she still alive?" I said she was in a nursing home in England and was in her mid-90s. He said, "We don't have much time." He asked Borlaug for a plan by the next morning! He proceeded to put in motion a plan that first demonstrated the value of the quality maize in the growth of pigs, and simultaneously began making the seeds available to farmers.

A few years later, in 1992, at the time of Williams's death, Borlaug reported that 60% of corn being planted in Ghana was now quality maize. His team was able to show an improvement in the nutritional status of children living in villages using the new variety.

This is one of many health improvements President Carter was able to introduce to Africa. Another fruitful pursuit of the Carter Center was its study designed to assess probable changes in the world's population, natural resources, and environment, as well as an appraisal of the ability of the government to respond to such changes. This resulted in the online publication, *The Global 2000 Report to the President: Entering the Twenty-First Century.*[6]

Faith Groups' Role in the United States

But President Carter also continued to seek ways of improving health in *this* country.

Faith groups had long felt an obligation to assist in promoting health, as reported in our chapter 5. They developed hospitals and clinics. The names of the original sponsors are still seen in the names of hospitals (e.g., St. Mary's hospital; Baptist, Presbyterian, or Lutheran hospitals), even if those hospitals are no longer run by faith groups. Over the years, these hospitals were purchased by for-profit groups. Faith groups subsequently reduced their health work. Running a hospital is a one-way street: those hospitals will never be repurchased by not-for-profit religious groups.

But there are other health activities that faith groups *could* pursue. During the 20th century, the average life expectancy of Americans improved by seven hours a day—that is, seven hours each day for slightly over 36,500 days. This statistic is almost beyond belief. Much of this improvement was the result of millions of daily decisions by Americans using scientific knowledge. Cessation of smoking, improvements in diet, acceptance of exercise programs, reduction in alcohol intake, fewer fatal car crashes, the use of sunscreen, vaccines of all kinds, iodine in salt, folic acid in food products—these are just some of the science-based interventions used even by people who express anti-science beliefs.

Faith groups could, if they are willing, provide a tremendous service to health. They could sponsor Smokender programs, nutrition-education programs, exercise facilities, Alcoholics Anonymous meetings, prevention-education programs, day care services for working parents, plus programs to help people navigate the complex environment of medical care, insurance plans, and referral services.

With this in mind, the Carter Center sponsored a meeting October 25–27, 1989, to explore what faith groups could offer. The symposium brought together 200 participants, including Christian, Jewish, Islamic, and Native American religious leaders. It resulted in a published report, *The Church's Challenge in Health*, available online from the website *cartercenter.org*.[7]

The symposium was productive in providing ideas on how faith groups could promote full and healthy lives. It began an effort that resulted in the program being adopted by Emory University's Rollins School of Public Health as an academic pursuit.

There are perils in enlisting faith groups for cooperative efforts when they may differ significantly in religious beliefs. We made clear from the beginning that we were interested in ideas to improve health and would avoid doctrinal and religious beliefs. Despite such assurances, one donor withdrew funding just before the meeting because of concern that abortion would be discussed. It caused great anxiety in finding replacement funds so late in the planning. (Actually, the subject of abortion was never raised because the list of other activities suggested by participants was so extensive and consuming.) The Carter Center also produced a publication, *Faith & Health*, a collection of articles highlighting the convergence of faith and health.[8]

Another fruitful pursuit of the Carter Center was its study designed to assess probable changes in the world's population, natural resources, and the environment, as well as an appraisal of the ability of the government to respond to such changes. This resulted in another publication.[6]

Mental health problems are often neglected and yet the World Bank's introduction of disability-adjusted life years (DALYs) has shown the incredible suffering and cost of mental health conditions. Mrs. Carter continued an interest in the subject, which had developed as her husband ran for governor in Georgia. She continued that interest as first lady and then into the global health field during the Carter Center years. One example was a program to detect stress disorders in students in Liberia, following brutal civil strife. Village workers were trained in detection and treatment techniques, demonstrating once again that it is possible to combine the skills and knowledge garnered in rich countries for the benefit of low-income areas.

Inspiring Students

For over 35 years, President Carter taught at Emory University in almost all departments. He also conducted an annual town hall meeting with freshmen each year. All questions were allowed, and he provided thoughtful answers, gleaned from his lifetime of experiences in politics, agriculture, nuclear engineering, global health, art, writing, travel, and religious study. At the age of 98, President Carter was still providing inspiration to the Carter Center and thus to the world.

Concluding Thoughts

Political involvement is often hidden in a program, so its value is easily underestimated. A reasonable summary of political involvement is that it has not provided the benefits that it could have. But in the future, as President Carter's post-presidential involvement in global health made so clear, political involvement could be the single greatest asset to improved global health. This would depend upon global health workers becoming better at including politicians in every program now operating and at the beginning of any new programs being developed.

But politics is just one major historical influencer of global health. Among others are colonialism, the military, religion, academics, bilateral and multilateral organizations, nongovernmental organizations, philanthropy, and the pharmacologic industry. These subjects are examined in detail in subsequent chapters. Summary thoughts will be given after each chapter regarding the positive and negative aspects of the chapter subject and their importance to global health.

CHAPTER 3

The Legacy of Colonialism in Global Health

PAUL ELISH

In the mid-20th century, the independence of British, French, Portu-guese, and Belgian colonies in Africa seemed to signal the end of co-lonialism. For global health, this new post-colonial era presented an opportunity to move beyond colonial paradigms. In reality, colonial paradigms remained (and remain) engrained in global health institu-tions and initiatives. There are many ways to decolonize global health, but none are promising if we don't first comprehend global health's colonial origins. Understanding the colonial roots of global health begins with understanding disease dynamics that date to Columbus's voyages across the Atlantic.

Hispaniola: A Case Study in Disease Dynamics after 1492

When Jean-Jacques Dessalines proclaimed the independence of the Haitian Republic from France on January 1, 1804, he sent shock waves through the global political order. Dessalines was born enslaved but proved himself an adept commander during the tumult of the Haitian Revolution.[1] Just as Dessalines's life story embodied a personal tri-umph over slavery, Haiti's independence represented a triumph of enslaved peoples that deeply disturbed colonial and slaveholding pow-ers in Europe, the United States, and elsewhere in the Americas.

The Haitian Revolution also represented a culmination of changing global disease dynamics. From the arrival of Christopher Columbus in the Caribbean three centuries earlier to the declaration of Haitian independence, the world underwent massive shifts in the distribution of disease. These disease shifts had a particularly striking impact on the history of Hispaniola, home to modern Haiti and the Dominican Republic. When we look at the history of disease in Hispaniola, we see a case study for how racism—particularly related to differing mortality rates across races—was at the core of colonial global health.

Race-related disease patterns became a central theme in Hispaniola's history when the Spanish arrived at the end of the 15th century. The Spanish conquest of the Caribbean was apocalyptic for the native Taíno people on Haití, their original name for the island now called Hispaniola.[2] Historians estimate that Hispaniola's native population was halved annually in the first years following initial contact with Europeans in the 1490s. By 1508, the Taíno population was approximately 60,000; in 1514, it had plummeted to 30,000, and by 1518, only 11,000 survived.[3] The population collapse was partially attributable to violence from colonizing Europeans, demands of forced labor, and disruptions in the food supply. It was also attributable to the sudden onslaught of diseases from Europe, Asia, and Africa to which the Indigenous populations had no immunity. Smallpox was the most devastating disease for native populations, but bubonic plague, influenza, malaria, measles, yellow fever, and typhus all had catastrophic consequences for native peoples as well. On Hispaniola, particularly fatal smallpox epidemics decimated the native population in 1518 and 1519. The Taíno population dwindled to a few hundred by 1570.[3]

While Indigenous populations suffered shattering mortality, Europeans initially considered the 16th-century Caribbean a paradise.[4] Nevertheless, European concerns about Indigenous mortality grew over time. Bartolomé de las Casas (1484–1566), a Dominican priest who initially possessed large tracts of land with enslaved Indigenous people before renouncing those holdings, became the most well-known Spanish defender of the native population. His 1520 account of Hispaniola noted how the Spanish were moved to stymie the Indigenous population's decline, primarily for economic reasons:

> A terrible plague came, and almost everyone died, very few remained alive. This was smallpox, which was given to the miserable Indians by some person from Castile . . . they die in a short time: adding to this are the weakness and hunger and the nudity and sleeping on the floor and overwork and the little health care that those they serve have always taken. Finally, the Spanish, seeing that the Indians were dying, began to feel the shortage (of labor), for which they moved to take some action to aid them, although it proved too little, because they should have begun it many years earlier; I do not believe that 1,000 souls escaped this misery, from the immensity of people that lived on this island and which we have seen with our own eyes.[5]

With Indigenous populations declining so rapidly, European colonists sought other sources of labor. The transatlantic slave trade gained momentum and brought millions of Africans to the Americas in bondage. Europeans had little idea that the slave trade would also transform the disease landscape in the Americas. Contrary to the initial European perception of the Caribbean as idyllic, Europeans in the mid-1700s had come to think of it as disease infested and lethal.[4] The main drivers of this change in perspective were yellow fever and malaria, which migrated across the Atlantic along with enslaved peoples.

Yellow fever could not have crossed the Atlantic in the body of an infected person since incubation and viremia total less than 10 days, which is shorter than the transatlantic voyage. Instead, yellow fever's migration probably happened because the mosquito *Aedes aegypti*'s eggs can survive for several months when desiccated. Desiccated mosquito eggs, inconspicuous on the slaving ships, would lay the foundation for a sea change in global disease dynamics.[6] Only a couple other ingredients were needed for yellow fever to establish solid footholds in the Caribbean: large human population reservoirs and time. The 17th-century sugar revolution, which established plantations in the eastern Caribbean, provided the necessary ingredients for outbreaks in the West Indies.[4]

Like yellow fever, malaria also used transatlantic voyages to leap to the Americas. It initially crossed the Atlantic in European sailors, but this first crossing had less consequence for Europeans since their immune systems were already primed for *Plasmodium vivax* and *P. malariae* species. In contrast, European immune systems were not prepared to fight the *P. falciparum* malaria species that was found in some African enslaved people. Africans who had falciparum immunity and Duffy negativity, which defended them against vivax malaria infections, were able to transport the falciparum species, which proved much deadlier for Europeans in the Americas. In some places like northeastern Brazil, falciparum malaria arrived as early as the 1500s on sugar plantations.[6] Falciparum malaria arrived in other places such as South Carolina much later, in the latter half of the 1600s.[7] During just a few centuries, the Caribbean had evolved from an area where immunity helped Europeans subjugate Indigenous peoples to a deadly region for European colonists.

The reversal in Europeans' disease susceptibility in the Caribbean laid the groundwork for major events in the Haitian Revolution. During the French Revolution in the 1790s, Haiti (then a French colony called Saint-Domingue) had gained considerable autonomy. In 1802, Napoleon sent an armada to Saint-Domingue with orders to bring the colony back under France's tight grip. The arrival of these French troops on the island launched the bloodiest period of the Haitian Revolution as the French and Haitians battled from February 1802 to November 1803.[1]

Jean-Jacques Dessalines was the main Haitian rebel leader in this period of intense fighting, and he was clear-eyed about the role of disease in the conflict. His exhortations to troops show just how much the Caribbean had changed since Bartolomé de las Casas had written his accounts nearly 300 years earlier:

> Have courage, have courage, I tell you, the French can't hold out
> long in Saint-Domingue. They will start off strongly, but soon they'll
> be slowed down by illness, and will die like flies. . . . They won't be
> able to hold the country, and they'll have to leave it.[1]

French forces initially won battles in Saint-Domingue, and many black Haitian generals (including Dessalines) defected to their side, but disease quickly reversed France's fortunes. By May 8, 1802—just three months after arriving in Saint-Domingue—only 12,000 of the initial 20,000 French troops remained for service. France's General Leclerc estimated that 200 to 250 French troops were falling ill each day. In June, a yellow fever epidemic blazed through the French forces while the Black population remained largely unscathed. The remaining French troops were far from sufficient to fully subjugate the colony.[1]

When news arrived, in August 1802, that Napoleon was reinstating slavery on other colonial islands, Haitian generals who had submitted to the French switched allegiances and launched a renewed insurrection. Leclerc observed the French forces' increasingly hopeless situation and suggested that a genocide against the island's Black population was the only way to regain control. Fortunately, Leclerc's suggestion was also thwarted. When Leclerc contracted yellow fever himself in November 1802 and died days later, France's renewal of war with Britain in spring 1803 doomed any hopes of reinforcements.[1] After the French surrendered in 1803, the victors named their new country Ayiti (Haiti) in honor of the island's original Amerindian Taíno people.[2] By that time, approximately 50,000 French military personnel had died, many at the hands of diseases that were not in the Americas 300 years previously.[1]

The "White Man's Grave" as Motivation for Colonial Global Health

The French experience in revolutionary Haiti reflected an increasingly clear pattern. Examples of European military catastrophes due to disease in the Caribbean stretched back to the mid-1600s. Among the English forces that seized Jamaica from Spain in 1655, some 5,000 out of 8,000 troops died of malaria and dysentery within one year.[7] British military forces experienced massive losses, again from yellow fever, during an expedition against the Spanish in modern-day Colombia in 1741 and yet again when moving against colonial Havana in 1762.[4]

The British Army surgeon stationed in Jamaica in 1782 reported that only 2,000 of the 7,000 British troops who had arrived in the previous three years were fit for duty.[3] The British, themselves, had tried to take Saint-Domingue in the 1790s, but by that time British troops in the Caribbean were dying from disease faster than they could be replaced. An estimated 80,000 British troops died in the Caribbean between 1793 and 1796; yellow fever alone accounted for more than half of those deaths.[4] The impact of disease also had consequences in civilian spheres. Of the 17,000 French settlers sent to colonize modern-day French Guiana in 1763, 60% died of dysentery, yellow fever, and malaria in a matter of months.[8] From the late 1600s through to the 19th century, yellow fever and falciparum malaria ensured there would be no large-scale European laborer population in the Caribbean.[7]

This pattern of high European mortality was not just seen in the Caribbean, and it continued in the 19th century. The West African coast was notoriously a "white man's grave," where disease, especially yellow fever and falciparum malaria, overwhelmed European attempts to explore the continent or create trading posts and plantations on the coast.[7,9] Europeans working in West Africa for the English Royal African Company (the English chartered slave-trading company) and its successor, the Company of Merchants Trading to Africa, experienced a mortality rate up to 391 deaths per 1,000 people per year from 1683 to 1766. This was comparable to the infant and child mortality rates of the era and far higher than the contemporary adult mortality rate. Europeans had a particularly high risk of death during the first six to eight months after arrival on the West African coast.[9] The pattern continued into the 19th century. In 1841–1842, the British Niger Expedition of 1841–1842 lost 350 per 1,000 people in under two months, and death tolls were also alarmingly high during British expeditions in Ethiopia and Ghana in the 1860s and 1870s.[4] In the mid-19th century, Britain recruited and trained West Africans as army medical officers because local West Africa populations appeared less susceptible to diseases that killed so many British personnel.[10]

By the mid-18th century, the tropics had acquired a persistently negative reputation in Europe. European writers noted a variety of dangers awaiting White men and women in the tropics, including catastrophic storms, vicious animals, and terrifying tropical diseases. European medical experts blamed warm and humid climates for poor European health in the tropics. The medical thinking of the era still favored Hippocrates and humoral theory, in which health was dictated by four humors: blood, black bile, yellow bile, and phlegm. These humors were differentiated by their hot-cold and wet-dry qualities—for example, blood was hot and moist while phlegm was cold and dry—and were thought to determine both physical and psychological health. With temperature and dryness being so fundamental to health, it made sense that hot, humid, tropical climates would harm Europeans who were accustomed to temperate environments. Many European observers concluded that Europeans were not biologically equipped to thrive in tropical settings. In 1818, British author James Johnson published *The Influence of Tropical Climates on European Constitutions* and voiced widely held pessimism about Europeans' ability to colonize and adapt to the climate in places like India.[11]

Given that Europeans considered environmental conditions the primary culprits for disease in the tropics, colonial solutions focused on colonists' immediate surroundings. Nineteenth-century British India provides a clear example of these environmental approaches to public health. When a large rebellion against British rule swept through India in 1857, epidemic diseases once again dramatically weakened British fighting capacity. Afterwards, the British created a commission to investigate the health of the British Army in India. In 1863, the Indian Royal Commission reported mortality among European troops to be 69 per 1,000 from 1800 to 1857, compared to 9 per 1,000 for British troops stationed in England. The findings were a scandal for the British public.[12]

With British troops' mortality unacceptably high, the 1864 military Cantonments Act was passed to improve hygiene in the troop barracks. Sanitary commissions and sanitary police were appointed to track and improve conditions in military camps.[12] Cholera was a source of substantial fear, and given its recently proven connection with water, many initiatives focused on improving drainage systems, water supplies, and cleaning systems for latrines. Some troops were also relocated to "hill stations," since higher elevations and cooler climates were deemed more amenable to European soldiers.[13]

Though British troops were the priority for sanitation improvements, it quickly became clear that military installations' sanitation did not operate in a vacuum. British administrators took offense at local populations' bazaars, villages, and religious spaces, whose sanitation was described as "remarkably objectionable." One British writer commented that "the natives of India have little or no idea of the value of sanitary arrangements. . . . The calls of nature are obeyed in the immediate vicinity of their villages and houses; no privies nor isolated localities are anywhere found."[13] British observers also criticized contaminated waterways at religious festivals and mismanaged livestock blood and waste at bazaars. Initial calls to separate military installations from local bazaars and other "contaminated" environments gave way to the realization that sanitation needed to be addressed in British cantonments and surrounding Indian communities to achieve lasting results. By the 1890s, British colonial authorities recognized that poor sanitation in Indian communities reduced British India's productivity and called for improved sanitation far beyond military enclaves.[13]

The Disregard for Non-White Mortality in Colonial Global Health

The colonial prioritization of White mortality could create the illusion that Indigenous populations did not suffer from disease. For example, the characterization of West Africa as a "white man's grave" overlooks the fact that local populations could suffer high mortality rates despite having some advantageous immunity compared to Europeans. Oftentimes, colonial powers did not treat Indigenous illness as an urgent problem unless it impacted labor supply and economic productivity, as occurred under the Spanish in 16th-century Hispaniola.

This warped perception of non-White mortality is especially evident in the transatlantic slave trade. Differences in European and African mortality from yellow fever and malaria emboldened claims that

Africans were biologically different from Europeans and were more predisposed to endure a warm climate and harsh labor. By extension, racial hegemonies that subordinated Africans, including the institution of slavery, were considered justified on "biological" grounds.[7,8]

In reality, enslaved Africans died en masse during the voyage across the Atlantic and while living in bondage in the Americas. For example, in 19th-century Brazil, it was well known that certain illnesses specifically devastated enslaved Africans. The Santa Casa de Misericórdia in Rio de Janeiro—one of a network of Santa Casa hospitals for the poor that Portuguese Queen Leonor established in 1498 and that continue to operate as a charity in the present day—treated many enslaved patients. It witnessed high infant mortality due to diarrhea and high adult mortality from tuberculosis and a gastrointestinal disease known as *maculo* in the 1800s. Some illnesses were considered entirely intertwined with slavery, including *caquexia africana* ("African wasting"), which entailed compulsive eating of plaster or dirt, and *banzo*, a form of depression in enslaved people that was attributed to nostalgia for Africa. Nevertheless, despite the suffering of enslaved peoples in Brazil, a more common critique of slavery was that the importation of Africans was bringing new illnesses to the free Brazilian population.[14] From a colonial perspective, the importance of death and suffering depended heavily on the race of those afflicted.

The Emergence of Germ Theory

In the latter half of the 1800s, Europe experienced a period of rapid scientific advancement, particularly in bacteriology. The discoveries would have profound implications for global health. Louis Pasteur of France and Robert Koch of Germany were two of the leading scientific luminaries of the period. In the 1860s, Pasteur proved that microbial life could not exist in environments that had been sterilized and protected from contamination.[12] In 1876, Koch released his findings about the microorganism that causes anthrax. Koch eventually published his celebrated postulates in 1890, which outlined criteria for determining a causal relationship between microbes and disease.[15] Pasteur's and

Koch's discoveries catalyzed broader scientific advances. From 1873 to 1888, scientists identified the bacterial pathogens for a slew of diseases, including gonorrhea, leprosy, typhoid fever, pneumonia, tuberculosis, cholera, diphtheria, tetanus, meningitis, and salmonellosis.[16] Pasteur and Koch also made pioneering attempts to develop vaccines, which contributed to a push to treat bacterial diseases with antitoxins and vaccination.[17]

These discoveries lent increasing strength to scientific medicine and related industries in Europe and the United States. Germany's renowned chemical industry, which initially focused on manufacturing dyes, gave birth to large pharmaceutical companies in the 1800s. Many of these companies, including Hoechst, Bayer, Ciba, Merck, and Sandoz, continue to exist either with their same name or as part of mergers in the present day. Germany's highly competitive university system also made the newly unified German Empire a medical research powerhouse that raced with French and British private and academic institutes to synthesize pharmaceuticals.[17]

Science was becoming a new forum for nationalist competition.[18] This contributed to the rise of "tropical medicine" and its associated academic institutions. The Liverpool School of Tropical Medicine and the London School of Tropical Medicine were founded in 1898 and 1899, respectively, while Portugal, France, Belgium, and the Netherlands founded schools in the 10 years that followed.[19]

Colonies were not left out of these scientific rivalries. Increasingly, the quest to dominate the colonial chessboard included the need for colonial powers to prove that they had the medico-scientific prowess to guarantee the health of their subjects, including Indigenous peoples in their colonial possessions.[17] Diverging scientific approaches led colonial powers to prioritize different health interventions in colonial settings.

Sleeping Sickness: Colonial Global Health Competition in the Age of Germ Theory

Sleeping sickness provides one of the clearest examples of European powers' competition and contrasting scientific visions in their colonies.[19] Human African trypanosomiasis, or sleeping sickness, is a parasitic disease that causes joint pain, headaches, fever, drowsiness, and swelling of lymph nodes at the back of the neck. Upon entering the central nervous system, the pathogens cause a person to become lethargic or psychotic and eventually comatose. The disease invariably leads to death, if left untreated, though those infected can survive for months or years, depending on whether they are infected with *Trypanosoma brucei gambiense* (which causes a more chronic disease) or *T. b. rhodesiense* (which kills sufferers within 12 months).[19]

Sleeping sickness was endemic in Africa for centuries before the heyday of European colonialism in the late 19th century. Nevertheless, colonial disruptions triggered an increase in epidemics that would lead to a range of responses from colonial powers that historian Daniel Headrick details in "Sleeping Sickness Epidemics and Colonial Responses in East and Central Africa, 1900–1940."[19] French and Belgian colonial activities in modern Congo-Brazzaville, Central African Republic, and the Democratic Republic of the Congo (DRC) increased mobility across local communities. Starting in the late 1880s, this increased movement led to outbreaks of sleeping sickness. In some cases, 20% of the population was infected. From 1901 to 1905, one-third of the population on Uganda's Lake Victoria shoreline died of sleeping sickness under British rule. In the years that followed, outbreaks also hit the British colonies in modern Sudan, Zambia, and Malawi, as well as the German colony in present-day Tanzania.[19]

European powers had economic, humanitarian, and prestige-related motives for addressing sleeping sickness, and scientists set to work understanding the disease. In this case, British researchers led the way. In 1895, David Bruce from the British Army Medical Service discovered the pathogen that caused nagana (the animal equivalent of human sleeping sickness) in the blood of horses and cattle. Bruce conclusively identified the protozoan *T. gambiense* as the cause of sleeping sickness in 1903, and his team of British researchers showed that tsetse flies living near rivers and lakes transmitted the disease. From 1901 onward, Portugal, Belgium, Germany, and France all sponsored their own investigations into sleeping sickness in colonial Africa.[19]

As Headrick explains, the different colonial powers pursued contrasting strategies for controlling sleeping sickness, based on their scientific arsenals and perspectives. The British favored an "environmental" approach that sought to separate colonial subjects from tsetse flies. In 1906, all Africans in Uganda were ordered to move out of areas within two miles of Lake Victoria because the lakeshore was considered a primary breeding ground for tsetse flies. Colonial authorities also banned fishing, the sale or possession of fish, gathering firewood, and hunting in the lakeshore zones. Sleeping sickness deaths fell under the new rules.[19]

Germany, in contrast to Britain, favored the use of pharmaceuticals, given German leadership in drug manufacturing. In the parts of modern Tanzania bordering Lake Victoria, German medical personnel trained local young men to identify villagers with swollen lymph glands and bring them to a camp for treatment with Atoxyl, a medication that frequently caused blindness but also showed promise as a treatment for sleeping sickness.[19]

European powers' colonial health decisions were also influenced by pressure to prove their ability to manage colonies. As the poorest of the colonizing countries, Portugal knew it did not have the resources to address sleeping sickness in its larger colonies of Angola and Mozambique. Instead, the Portuguese decided to demonstrate their public health capacities by waging a war of attrition against sleeping sickness on the small island of Príncipe. Beginning in 1911, prisoners from other Portuguese colonies were brought to Príncipe to drain swamps and clear land associated with tsetse flies. Wild pigs, civet cats, monkeys, and stray dogs were all hunted and killed because of their suspected roles as reservoirs for the disease. All Príncipe inhabitants were given Atoxyl, the sick were isolated in camps, and villagers were relocated from tsetse-infested areas. The percentage of infected inhabitants plummeted from 26% in 1907 to less than 1% in 1914.[19]

France similarly felt pressure to address sleeping sickness. When the French took over the German colony of Cameroon after World War I, the German press accused the French of neglecting Cameroonian subjects' health. Eugène Jamot, the director of the Pasteur Institute in the

French Congo and the leader of French efforts against sleeping sickness, instituted a system of mobile medical teams that roved from village to village and administered Atoxyl to the sick. France successfully overcame repeated sleeping sickness outbreaks by the late 1930s, but its singular focus on sleeping sickness left other major endemic diseases unaddressed. Both the Portuguese and French initiatives against sleeping sickness illustrate how political considerations could shape colonial health strategy more than disease burden. Portugal and France saw sleeping sickness as a high-profile disease, and they were eager to win praise by fighting it even if this meant ignoring larger colonies or other diseases.[19]

Yet the most consistent theme in the colonial campaigns against sleeping sickness was a disregard for colonial subjects' culture, input, and general welfare. The British relocation orders and fishing bans successfully reduced sleeping sickness deaths, but they introduced new hardships for Ugandans, who previously farmed on the lakeshore and relied on fish for protein. In German-held Tanzania, villagers began resisting the sleeping sickness initiatives because they suspected that Atoxyl treatment was worse than the disease itself. The French readily used coercion at gunpoint to administer Atoxyl, and it became common for colonial subjects to hide in the forest upon hearing that France's mobile sleeping sickness teams were approaching.[19]

The Belgian Congo provides an example of an even more authoritarian approach to colonial health. Communities with tsetse fly infestations were sealed off via *cordons sanitaires*, and locals were required to carry medical passports to travel any farther than a short distance from home.[20] Those infected were sent to camps and injected with Atoxyl. Locals dreaded these sleeping sickness camps because of the poor conditions, malnutrition, and loneliness awaiting detainees, and soldiers had to guard the camps to prevent escapes.[19]

These authoritarian measures against sleeping sickness were consistent with racialized authoritarian health measures that Belgium established more broadly in the Congo. In 1898, a segregation decree separated cities into White and Black zones to reduce "contamination" across races; in Belgian Leopoldville, Africans were not allowed in the

White zone from 9 p.m. to 6 a.m. unless they had a special pass.[20] Britain, Germany, and France all similarly considered racial segregation an effective strategy against diseases such as malaria in their colonies.[7]

The Belgian Congo also demonstrates the limits of authoritarian approaches to public health programs.[19] Belgium was consistently concerned about declining labor from low African birth rates and high mortality in the Congo. This led colonial authorities to pursue comprehensive health programs like that of the Kilo-Moto Gold Mine in the present-day Democratic Republic of the Congo's northeast. By the 1950s, the mining company offered free medical care to workers and surrounding villagers, and its technicians and medical staff addressed water management, waste disposal, malaria control, and housing. Yet Congolese workers generally disliked and avoided the housing, toilets, and potable water associated with the mine because they were "imposed by an uninvited and unwelcome authority, without local consultation."[20]

Colonial Public Health as Propaganda

Colonialism was frequently justified based on the "gifts" that were brought to colonial subjects, such as Western medicine, infrastructure, and education. Scientific and medical advances in Europe and the United States in the late 1800s gave colonizing powers more confidence that they were doing a service for colonized peoples. Medicine was an especially powerful tool for colonial administrations seeking to win legitimacy. French political scientist and historian Olivier Le Cour Grandmaison explores France's use of medicine for colonial propaganda in L'Empire des hygiénistes: faire vivre aux colonies.[8] Like other colonizing powers, French colonial authorities came to recognize medical services as a propaganda tool by the beginning of the 20th century. In 1907, Drs. Edmond and Étienne Sergent wrote that "the doctor is the European who inspires the most confidence in the indigenous person, who is admitted everywhere, who makes himself heard, and whom all obey without him having to resort to force." In essence, healthcare made for excellent public relations that could win over the hearts of colonized communities and legitimize conquest.[8]

With this strategy in mind, French forces placed heavy emphasis on "native medical assistance" during campaigns in Madagascar and Morocco. During these expeditions, medical outreach was given precedence over military maneuvers. As Olivier Le Cour Grandmaison writes, French weapons and medical care were "two faces of one enterprise that would serve the stability of overseas territories and finally solidly establish French sovereignty [in those territories]."[8]

Medical outreach in the French colonies also served as good propaganda on the home front. Publications directed at the French public and French students emphasized France's medical services in Africa and Asia to illustrate how French colonialism was uniquely focused on "collaboration and friendship." Victor Hugo himself praised the new age of colonialism in 1879, arguing that the French Republic's colonial mission emancipated Africans through the "plow," "commerce," and "industry," in contrast to previous colonial ventures that simply served the whims of despots.[8]

As French physician Dr. Jules Colombani wrote in 1927, France was concerned with "making [the Indigenous people] benefit" since they represented "brothers and humanity less privileged than [the French]." Yet self-interested motives were never far beneath the surface. Like in 16th-century Hispaniola, the health of conquered populations affected the labor supply in France's new possessions. Dr. Colombani himself admitted that the medical outreach also served utilitarian purposes because it could "conserve by all means possible the local human capital for maximally complete workforce output, which is needed from the very first day for the development of the newly occupied country."[8]

Colonialism as a Cause of Public Health Disasters

Colonial efforts to construe healthcare outreach as a gift to the colonized were largely disingenuous since healthcare also had the motive of preserving the labor force. Even more importantly, the idea of colonial administrations improving health was often misleading since colonialism frequently created or exacerbated health issues. Sleeping sickness provides one example. As previously described, the increased mobility associated with French and Belgian colonialism in central Africa seeded large epidemics of sleeping sickness.

Colonial India provides other striking examples of the health-related perils of colonialism. India experienced 20 famines between 1860 and 1910. The most severe was the Great Famine of 1876–1878. It was precipitated by El Niño–related shifts in rainfall, but it was exacerbated by new colonial economic conditions. Before British rule, Indians dealt with recurring famines through grain stores managed by local princes and moguls.[21] In contrast, British administrators worried that distributing food directly to the population would diminish the population's work ethic. Instead, the British chose a laissez-faire approach that relied on market forces to ensure adequate food supply, or they opted to provide relief in exchange for labor on public infrastructure projects such as railroads and irrigation construction. India had relatively high agricultural productivity leading up to the drought of 1876, but the opening of the Suez Canal in 1869 and expanding railroads diverted much of the bounty to England. Local food reserves that traditionally buffered against famine were drained, and the market's "invisible hand" brought no relief. Up to 8 million Indians died in the Great Famine that followed.[21]

The infrastructure projects the British favored for distributing "welfare" also had disastrous consequences. In the early 1880s, not long after the Great Famine had torn through Indian society, the British put Indian laborers to work digging 12,750 miles of irrigation canals. The new canals collected standing water and, as a result, mosquitoes' breeding opportunities expanded exponentially.[7] The canal project made India a tinderbox for colossal malaria epidemics. Malaria outbreaks erupted and devastated Indian communities, whose immune systems were already weakened by malnourishment from recent famines. There were opportunities for treatment (quinine had been known to treat malaria for centuries and was widely used globally), but the British reserved quinine for White colonials. Millions of Indians died as malaria surged through the population.[7] This pattern of colonialism sowing seeds for epidemics was not unique to British India. Across colonies controlled by various colonial powers, epidemics burst forth as a result of altered wildlife habitats, population migrations, changes in the food supply, and rapid urbanization associated with colonialism.[10]

The Power of Local Intermediaries and Subordinates in Colonial Global Health

Much of the scholarship on colonial health has focused on the influence and decisions of high-level colonial administrators. Previous sections in this chapter illustrate how administrators had sweeping power over local populations. Additionally, historical archives tell us far more about high-level administrators than about local subordinates, whose identities and activities were less frequently recorded. Nevertheless, as scholars have noted in more recent decades, the power of colonizing authorities over the local population was not always absolute. Local people sometimes held intermediary positions in the colonial hierarchy and could wield significant power over colonial public health practices.[10] Even though these individuals from colonized populations were below colonial administrators in the official hierarchy, implementation of public health initiatives could hinge on their buy-in and activities.

Historians of the British Empire have studied the power of intermediaries and subordinates especially thoroughly. In their 2012 volume *Public Health in the British Empire: Intermediaries, Subordinates, and the Practice of Public Health, 1850–1960*, coeditors Ryan Johnson and Amna Khalid call for a greater focus on how colonial subjects influenced colonial public health:

> Colonial officials were obliged to communicate with subject populations through intermediary and subordinate agents, not least because of barriers of language and culture. Yet the historiography of public health in the colonies has focused, with a few exceptions, on debates in the upper tiers of colonial sanitary and medical administrations.

These debates and professional rivalries in the process of policy making are important and have their place in the story of public health in colonial societies, but they do not capture the practice and implementation of public health policy on the ground. In addition, these accounts tend to portray colonial policy as the result of imperial exigencies and the interests of colonial administrators, overlooking the manner and degree to which agents on the ground were able to impact policy.[10]

Johnson, Khalid, and the scholars who contributed to their volume describe how British colonial public health was not always a "top-down process." In some cases, colonialism involved a process of negotiation in which local intermediaries had substantial agency. This was especially true because the British Empire employed indirect rule in South Asia and Africa, wherein day-to-day colonial administration was left to local and traditional rulers. As a result, the empire relied heavily on Indigenous subjects—including local rulers, interpreters, administrative clerks, soldiers, prison guards, businesspeople, domestic and agricultural workers, or healthcare personnel—to carry out colonial initiatives. After World War I, Britain transferred even more activities to local control, including public health and education initiatives, in an effort to cut costs and improve efficiency.[10]

Colonial administrations needed local leadership to overcome language barriers in public health. In the British colony of Burma, the increased local leadership in public health in the 1920s and 1930s improved public health propaganda initiatives. Burmese public health officials created health pamphlets, articles, posters, magic lantern slides, lectures, and films in the local vernacular.[22]

In one of its most ambitious and successful health communications projects, the new Burmese Department of Public Health outfitted a train carriage with health-related charts and models. An entirely Burmese team of three sub-assistant surgeons, two nurses, and two clerks rode with the train and educated the public. A separate "cinema carriage" allowed the Department of Public Health to hold screenings of health films in local languages as the train traveled to 20 towns in rural Burma. An average of 5,000 people visited the train daily, and an estimated 1,500 people watched the screenings each night during the 23-day tour. These activities, grounded in local languages, had not been possible when British colonial administrators dictated public health messaging.[22]

In other cases, local leaders could leverage colonial public health for their own interests. When plague arrived in colonial Ghana in 1908, the British Colonial Office feared that the outbreak would sweep through the entire colony. Instead, only about 300 people died. The successful containment was largely thanks to a local leader in Accra, Kojo Ababio, who organized laborers to hunt rats, destroy infected houses, and evacuate part of the capital. Ababio used the evacuation as a pretense for settling his people on valuable contested land outside Accra (to the chagrin of other local groups), and his cooperation with colonial authorities won him and his people significant funding to build housing.[23]

In other cases, colonial public health was entirely beholden to local populations. In colonial India, members of low castes were responsible for scavenging and sweeping, including the collection and disposal of human waste at night. These "sweepers" had a hereditary right to control sanitation for particular private households and neighborhoods and were paid with food, clothes, or money from the served households. Additionally, the colonial state sometimes relied on sweepers to report deaths because sweepers' sanitation duties gave them enhanced access to private residences. This surveillance responsibility became especially important during epidemics. In one 1896 bubonic plague outbreak, dead bodies were hidden from government officials because local populations perceived autopsies as a desecration of the deceased. In response, the government paid sweepers to report plague deaths to track the epidemic.[24]

Sweepers, because they respected each other's hereditary holdings, functioned as a form of unofficial workers union. If a household lodged a complaint against a hereditary sweeper, sweepers would often boycott the complaining house. Sweepers went on strike repeatedly, including in 1873, 1876, and 1889 in Delhi and twice in 1889 in Bombay. During the strikes, city hygiene became unbearable, and public health authorities feared outbreaks of diseases. The colonial administration wanted to abolish customary sweeping and create a system of municipally employed sweepers that it could more directly control, but the sweepers had substantial collective power. Colonial administrators left the traditional system in place for fear of the sweepers' reaction to changes.[24]

In many instances, British colonial authorities tried and failed to replace local healing practices with Western medicine. In modern-day Chennai, India, in the late 19th century, the British trained local women as midwives to replace the *dais*, the traditional birth attendants, who had no formal medical education. The fact the trainings were initially conducted in English meant that only mission-educated Christians were eligible. However, Christian midwives were suspect to the general population because their religion placed them outside the traditional social order. Even when the British relented and established midwifery trainings in local languages to attract non-Christian recruits, dais remained widely used because the British-trained midwives were never trained to communicate the merits of midwifery to the general populace. In cases in which Indian families called trained midwives, they often did so when also calling a dai; the midwife could be present at the birth, but families still wanted a dai to control the birthing process.[25]

The British similarly struggled to shape local beliefs and practices in African colonies. In present-day Zambia from the 1940s to the 1950s, the Christian Missions in Many Lands (CMML) medical missionary organization trained medical auxiliaries in Western medicine with support from the British colonial government. Traditionally, the local Lunda tribe viewed illness as a product of dysfunctional social relationships and believed healers had to repair kinship relationships to address sickness. CMML viewed this traditional understanding of disease as a barrier to Christian conversion and sought to weaken it by training locals in Western medicine.[26]

Yet social disruption in colonial Zambia actually strengthened traditional beliefs and associated healing practices. At the time, inequality was rising. The British were investing heavily in copper mining, and some farmers became rich by growing crops for the burgeoning copper mine workforce. The new wealth sowed division in rural families, and it became common to accuse newly rich relatives of using witchcraft to accrue wealth. The local population expected medical auxiliaries to heal in the traditional sense, including serving as arbiters for family disputes. However, CMML had limited success in changing these expectations. Despite its opposition, medical auxiliaries incorporated locally inspired healing rituals into their work, including overnight prayer vigils, in which auxiliaries protected against witchcraft and encouraged relatives to resolve disputes with the sick.[26]

Colonialism and the Rise of Global Organizations

Multilateral organizations, or organizations formed by three or more countries for collaboration purposes, play a large role in present-day global health. The most prominent modern multilaterals, including the United Nations (UN), the World Health Organization (WHO), and the World Bank, arose in the middle of the 1900s as the world recovered from World War II. The new postwar multilateralism quickly threatened colonial powers, who wanted to avoid international interference in their colonies. But international collaboration was not new. By the mid-20th century, international cooperation in global health had already existed for almost 100 years.

Technological advances and colonialism were driving forces for international collaboration in the 1800s. New technology for trains and steamships left the world more interconnected, and colonialism linked far-flung parts of the globe. Growing global trade further connected continents. The increased trade and interconnectivity created a need for greater standardization of regulations across countries. Whereas only 24 international meetings of any size or purpose were held from 1800 to 1850, some 1,390 international meetings transpired from 1851 to 1899. New organizations such as the International Telegraphic Union (founded in 1865), the Universal Postal Union (founded 1874), and the Union of Weights and Measures (1875) answered the call for standardization. The 19th century's scientific advances also gave rise to scientific congresses to share discoveries.[18]

This increased connectivity also gave diseases opportunities to spread more quickly. Cholera was the most prominent disease to rocket around the globe in the 1800s. After originating in South Asia's Ganges River Delta, cholera expanded in a series of five 19th-century pandemics. The second pandemic began in 1829 and reached Europe and North America in the 1830s before subsiding around 1851. By the 1850s, European medical professionals agreed that future outbreaks could not be stopped if countries acted unilaterally. In an effort to standardize cholera quarantine procedures, the first International Sanitary Conference was held in Paris in 1851; 12 countries sent delegations. Ten such conferences about cholera would take place from 1851 to 1900.[18] Eventually, the conferences gave rise to a formal multilateral organization, the International Office of Public Hygiene (*Office international d'hygiène publique*; OIHP).[27]

A core objective of the Sanitary Conferences was to protect Europe from future cholera outbreaks, but the incentive to collaborate in defense of Europe was often insufficient for action. Imperial rivalries, such as between France and Germany, hindered cooperation. Across conferences, there was also a consistent push to check Britain's geopolitical power through greater international control of sanitary measures, such as in Egypt near the Suez Canal. The British resisted. When a Sanitary Conference tried to impose rules on British India, British delegates responded, "India ought not to be fettered or cramped by any International Convention." Britain wielded enough power to outright refuse to cooperate and end conferences, as it did in 1885 in response to the Suez Canal debates.[18]

A more dangerous precedent was set by the conferences' double standard on quarantines. European military ships were not subjected to any controls, even though they posed a high risk for spreading cholera. Instead, delegates focused heavily on Muslim pilgrims to Mecca. The pilgrims were already viewed with suspicion by Western observers, so it was not a far leap to categorize them as a public health threat. One British delegate remarked on the risk of this double standard in

1894, noting that Muslim pilgrims had only introduced cholera in Europe once, whereas European military operations in present-day Afghanistan had brought cholera to Europe several times.[18] The colonial powers' selective, discriminatory commitment to multilateral health measures undermined multilateralism's effectiveness. Even after the OIHP was formed, it had little real power beyond sharing epidemiologic information.[27]

This fraught relationship between colonialism and multilateralism had consequences decades later. In the 1940s, colonial powers, including France, viewed the newly formed UN and WHO with trepidation. Historian Jessica Pearson analyzes this phenomenon in the context of France in *The Colonial Politics of Global Health: France and the United Nations in Postwar Africa*.[27] Internally, French officials worried that these new international organizations would rival France's expertise in its own colonies and commit it to costly long-term development projects. French diplomats also expressed concern about how anticolonial delegations would use the UN as a venue to highlight colonial health and social problems, and they feared that international organizations' representatives would come to the colonies and open them to international criticism. In many respects, these fears came to fruition: anti-imperialist UN delegations soon pointed at poor living standards in colonies as evidence of injustice. The UN charter itself instructed colonial governments to support colonies' efforts toward self-government.[27]

Colonizing countries used various approaches to overcome the growing criticism. Britain devolved various powers to local authorities. France took the unique step of creating the "French Union" in 1946, which theoretically made colonial subjects equal citizens with those French living in Europe. France was aiming to make Africans more French at the same time that delegations from newly independent countries like India and Indonesia aimed to promote self-determination through the UN. French officials hoped their approach would shield France from criticism in a global environment that was steadily becoming more anticolonial.[27]

Colonial powers also proactively resisted multilateralism in global health. The establishment of WHO's regional offices became a sticking point. France tried and failed to get French North Africa included in WHO's European Region in an effort to tie its North African colonies' identity to Europe. Belgian, British, and French colonial officials all schemed to stop WHO from establishing a regional office in Africa, since they feared a WHO Africa Office would open their African colonies to more direct criticism. As part of this effort, the three colonial powers created collaborative organizations with the idea that they would make a WHO regional office in Africa unnecessary. The Commission for Technical Cooperation in Africa South of the Sahara (*Commission de coopération technique en Afrique au sud du Sahara*; CCTA) was formed in 1949 and the International Children's Centre (*Centre international de l'enfance*; CIE) was founded in 1950. Belgium, Britain, and France argued that they already fulfilled the role of a regional office.[27]

This colonial resistance to multilateralism had several consequences. The WHO Regional Office for Africa was the last WHO regional office established, even though Africa had a clear need for international assistance. The resistance of colonial governments in Africa also contributed to the notorious failure of WHO's Malaria Eradication Program (MEP, 1953–1969).[27]

In 1950, WHO and CCTA held a joint conference in Uganda to discuss the potential for a coordinated antimalaria campaign. After that conference, colonial governments embarked on their own pilot programs against malaria. France's antimalaria programs faced financial constraints, and France turned to the UN, WHO, and UNICEF for financial assistance. France and WHO were soon at odds over the assistance that WHO would provide.[27]

The main source of disagreement was a WHO rule requiring that only 25% of technical assistance funds be given for materials, such as DDT, house-spraying equipment, and transport vehicles. WHO instead dedicated most funding to supplying experts and technical personnel—precisely the assistance France did *not* want. French colonial administrators were reluctant to let non-French UN experts advise on malaria in French Africa since foreign experts could undermine France's scientific and medical justification for its colonial presence. The French delegation at the first annual meeting of the WHO Regional Committee for Africa argued that technical expertise was already sufficient in most African territories, so WHO should just provide funding and supplies for the existing colonial antimalaria campaigns. Internally, French officials discussed ways to ensure that WHO experts would only be present before and after antimalaria campaigns to assess progress, rather than providing direct technical support.[27]

With time, French efforts to keep WHO experts out of its antimalaria campaigns were hobbled by rising malaria morbidity and mortality in France's colonies. WHO and the French colonial administration compromised, and WHO shouldered a bigger financial burden for antimalarial efforts than initially projected. Nevertheless, the delayed cooperation hurt MEP's scale-up. Colonial resistance to international collaboration on malaria was one factor in MEP's overall failure, alongside its broader failure to account for local cultural practices and preferences.[27]

Colonialism's Long Shadow in Modern Global Health

Colonial global health evolved dramatically from the late 1400s to the mid-20th century. European anxieties about White mortality in the tropics, especially mortality among soldiers, brought health to the forefront in colonial ventures. Beliefs that White mortality in the tropics was caused by climate eventually gave way to germ theory in the late 19th century, which shifted the blame to microorganisms and their human carriers. Colonizing powers, once they determined that Indigenous peoples' health should be preserved for labor and propaganda purposes, stopped disregarding Indigenous peoples' mortality. In the meantime, colonial disruptions caused recurring disasters for Indigenous health. By the early 1900s, colonial health initiatives targeting Indigenous populations were frequently authoritarian in nature, even as local intermediaries managed to exert power in some cases. By the mid-20th century, the fading colonial era still had implications for new multilateral global health entities.

In the 21st century, the colonial era can seem distant. The more extreme colonial global health abuses described in this chapter are no longer commonplace. Nevertheless, the patterns and practices of colonial global health can still be identified in modern global health. The colonial tendency to impose top-down solutions while downplaying input from local communities has not entirely disappeared. Championing technical Western medical interventions over social determinants of health remains a common paradigm. Even more common is the tendency of power imbalances, international economics, and geopolitical interests to shape global health activities carried out by militaries, bilateral organizations, academic institutions, and other actors. In the chapters that follow, the echoes of the colonial era remind us of the continued need to decolonize global health.

Concluding Thoughts
BILL FOEGE

Colonialism employed a spectrum of approaches, but power and greed were the drivers. The shared ingredient was one country co-opting another. The benefits were often said to be the introduction of science, technology, religion, business, and better health and management skills to an area that had not benefited from modern developments.

These benefits are clear in irrigation systems in the subcontinent, efficient trains in India, and improved transportation systems around the world. Globalism was one of the lasting contributions.

But the price was exceedingly high. Deaths, suffering, poverty, and social disruption far outweigh any benefits attributed to colonialism. Slavery and its aftermath are constant reminders that society will pay for centuries in the future when the avarice of strong countries leads them to impose their will on weak areas of the world. The deaths and disruption from smallpox and other plagues far exceed any medical benefits brought to Africa, Asia, and the Americas.

Colonialism is a given and can't be reversed, but the harm needs to be acknowledged. Tragedy triumphed.

CHAPTER 4

Militaries and Global Health

PAUL ELISH

In 1899, a ship traveling from Hong Kong brought bubonic plague to Manila. The Philippines had only recently become a colony of the United States, but as historian Warwick Anderson describes in *Colonial Pathologies: American Tropical Medicine, Race, and Hygiene in the Philippines*,[1] the colonial administration took rapid action through the Manila Board of Health. Docking ships were inspected for infected passengers and rodents, the sick were quarantined, sickrooms were disinfected, clothing of the sick was burned, and the public was encouraged to only drink boiled water. Over the years that followed, health authorities pursued a crusade against rats. Ratcatchers targeted the most heavily affected neighborhoods and transported 20,000 rats to a government laboratory in February 1902 alone; the lab found 13 infected rats after inspecting 10,000 under microscopes. That same year, the Philippines was rocked by a cholera outbreak, and similarly strong measures were taken. The sick were brought to a centralized tent hospital, board of health officers went from house to house to find cases and confiscate food that was deemed infected, members of infected households were forcibly bathed in a bichloride solution, and sanitary inspectors and the cavalry joined forces to restrict access to the Marikina River, where many residents normally retrieved water.[1]

Such tactics did help reduce the burden of bubonic plague and cholera, and both epidemics ended by 1906. Yet local attitudes about the public health interventions were not entirely positive. Even though poor Filipinos bore the brunt of cholera, many tried to hide cholera cases because US health interventions were associated with property destruction and painful experimental treatments. Many Filipinos were prepared to take loved ones into the rice fields at night rather than turn them over to cholera detention camps. One wealthier Filipino, Dr. T. H. Pardo de Tavera, informed Governor William Taft that "the people fear the Board of Health a great deal more than they fear the epidemic."[1]

It comes as no surprise that US colonial health policies in the Philippines were heavily influenced by military culture, given that the United States had seized the Philippines in the Spanish-American War. What seems to have surprised American colonial health authorities was the dual effect of a militarized approach to public health: Although aggressive public health measures could stamp out some outbreaks and tighten control over the population, they simultaneously alienated local communities and jeopardized public health campaigns in the long term. In the case of cholera, American colonial health authorities changed course and allowed the sick to isolate at home. American health officials in the Philippines came to realize that a more conciliatory approach with local populations could benefit public health campaigns in the years that followed.[1]

The experience of American colonial public health in the Philippines illustrates some of the broader contradictions of military involvement in global health. This chapter explores the role of militaries in global health in additional depth, tracking military involvement from the naval origins of tropical medicine to contemporary military global health activities, with a particular focus on trends in the United States. Though global health has changed substantially in the past two centuries, connections to militaries and broader notions of defense have remained strong. These military connections can have both positive and negative consequences.

The Naval Origins of Global Health

Sir Patrick Manson is traditionally considered the "father of tropical medicine" for his groundbreaking research on mosquito-borne disease and his role in founding the London School of Hygiene & Tropical Medicine (LSHTM). Despite this fame, he had humble roots. Born in a small town north of Aberdeen, Scotland, he served as an apprentice to ironmasters until a case of vertebral tuberculosis left him bedridden as a teenager. The bout of tuberculosis also fatefully changed his career path. After recovering, he became a medical student at the University of Aberdeen, and he was appointed as a physician for the Chinese Maritime Customs Service (a tax collection agency in China) after graduation. It was in Asia that Manson built his reputation as an expert in the emerging field of tropical medicine. In the 1870s, he conducted pioneering experiments in China that showed the man–mosquito transmission pathway for elephantiasis. He founded LSHTM (then known simply as the London School of Tropical Medicine) in 1899.[2]

Patrick Manson's decision to begin his medical career in a maritime customs organization led to an enduring link between him and naval medicine. He spent five years inspecting ships in modern-day Taiwan when he started working for the Chinese Maritime Customs Service. He then spent 13 years working in present-day Xiamen in mainland China, where he oversaw a hospital for European seamen. He also conducted his groundbreaking research on elephantiasis during this period and contributed to the Medical Reports of the Imperial Maritime Customs, writing about diseases seen in Xiamen. Upon returning to England, Manson worked at Albert Dock Seamen's Hospital in London and at Greenwich's Dreadnought Hospital. In both cases, he treated sailors with diseases acquired on voyages abroad. It was thus no accident that Manson designated Albert Dock Seaman's Hospital as the site for training medical officers destined for West Africa when he was appointed Medical Officer of the Colonial Office in 1897, and as the first site of the London School of Tropical Medicine in 1899.[2]

The recurring theme of naval medicine in Patrick Manson's life reflects broader trends in early global health. Before the scientific advances of the late 19th century, British naval surgeons were considered to have the most expertise on "exotic" diseases, given that they treated sailors on voyages around the globe.[1] In France before Louis Pasteur, "colonial medicine" was the domain of the French navy, and its main practitioners were concentrated in the French ports of Brest, Rochefort, and Toulon.[3] It was not until 1890 that France established a colonial health corps separate from its naval medical division. Even after that change, most French doctors in the colonies came from the military because of insufficient civilian recruits.[4]

The United States Public Health Service provides another example of the naval roots of many public health and global health institutions. In 1797, a US congressional committee reported that many seamen were arriving at US ports in very poor health, overburdening existing hospitals, and dying from a lack of appropriate care. In response, US President John Adams established "marine hospitals" in 1798 to care for sick and disabled merchant seamen (and initially members of the US Navy, though a separate naval hospital system was established in 1811).[5] Over the course of its history, the system of marine hospitals gave birth to an array of American institutions. The Boston Marine Hospital became the first teaching hospital in the United States when Harvard medical students began instructional sessions on its medical wards in 1807. A small bacteriology laboratory set up in an attic at the Staten Island Marine Hospital in 1887 was transferred to Washington, DC, in 1891 and grew to be the National Institutes of Health. Later, after World War I, the marine hospitals were tasked with caring for injured and disabled veterans and expanded to operate 81 hospitals. Within two years, the "Veteran's Bureau" took over the administration of 57 of these hospitals as the modern Veterans Administration (VA) took shape.[5]

The military roots of the marine hospitals were also reinforced over time. In 1871, marine hospitals were transferred from local to federal control because of alleged mismanagement. During this reorganization, the marine hospitals were placed under Dr. John Woodworth, who was named the "Supervising Surgeon of the Marine Hospital Service (MHS)." This role would eventually become the modern-day

Surgeon General.[5] While at the helm of the MHS, Dr. Woodworth instituted a military model for medical staff. Later, in 1889, the US Congress formally established the United States Public Health Service Commissioned Corps within the MHS, which created a structure of titles and pay scales that mimicked army and navy systems.[6]

The MHS's broadened mandate earned it a name change in 1912, becoming the US Public Health Service (USPHS). Meanwhile, the role of the marine hospitals (which had become "Public Health Service hospitals") shrank during the 20th century, especially with the growth of the VA. In 1981, all but one of the remaining 9 PHS hospitals and 27 PHS clinics ceased to operate.[5] Nevertheless, the USPHS Commissioned Corps remains in action and maintains its military model.

Global Health and Military Rivalry at the Turn of the Century

Global health also has roots in military rivalry. By the time the European "Scramble for Africa" began in the late 19th century, military health had become an arena for competition on a global scale. France felt a particularly urgent need to catch up with other European powers in the race to lower troops' mortality, as examined in Olivier Le Cour Grandmaison's *L'Empire des Hygiénistes: Faire Vivre aux Colonies*.[7] Dr. Gustave Reynaud, a leading French physician, estimated that French troops' mortality abroad reached as high as 74%, compared to less than 20% among British forces in India and the Caribbean.[7] Many French medical professionals admired the British emphasis on hygienic conditions for their colonial regiments, and the longstanding, relatively healthy British population in India inspired awe (and envy) in French circles.[7] With time, France also competed with Germany on colonial health. In 1903, French Dr. Paul Reille expressed dismay that French soldiers' mortality was "four times higher than in Germany," due to typhoid and tuberculosis.[7]

French doctors blamed high mortality rates on a colonial strategy that sidelined physicians and on military leaders who paid little heed to medical advice. The doctors expressed horror at ships that were overcrowded, poorly ventilated, and swelteringly hot; barracks that were poorly situated and unhygienic; long marches while carrying heavy loads; and arduous work in broad sunlight.[7] Above all, French medical personnel were unhappy with being locked out of colonial leadership and decision-making. One physician complained that the "doctor's place" in colonial expeditions was always in the "rear guard," where they were left to "collect the crippled," instead of serving as leaders. In the eyes of these physicians, a colonial doctor's proper place was alongside superior officers.[7]

Over time, the critiques brought change. From the 1890s onward, France sought to make science and health more central to its colonial administration. In 1890, "l'École principale du service de santé de la marine" (the Principal School of the Naval Health Service) opened its doors in Bordeaux to produce more doctors for colonial troops. A similar program was established for civilian doctors to study "colonial medicine" in 1896.[7] French nongovernment initiatives went even further than government initiatives. By 1910, France's great scientist Louis Pasteur had developed a network of Instituts Pasteur with centers in modern-day Vietnam, Senegal, Madagascar, Congo-Brazzaville, and Martinique. Dr. Alphonse Laveran, who won a Nobel Prize in medicine for his malaria-related discoveries, established the Exotic Pathology Society in 1908. This society quickly became a reputed research organization.[7] Rivalry with Britain and Germany had laid the groundwork for France's global health infrastructure.

The Spanish-American War and Yellow Fever

The United States's swift victory in the Spanish-American War in the 1890s gave the country a bigger role on the world's geopolitical stage. The war also led to deep US military involvement in health initiatives abroad, especially tied to yellow fever. While 400 American soldiers were killed in combat during the war's battles in the Caribbean and the Philippines, more than 2,000 American soldiers succumbed to yellow fever. After the war in 1900, Surgeon General George Sternberg sent a commission, led by Major Walter Reed, to investigate yellow fever and determine ways to reduce troop mortality.[8]

There were already suspicions that mosquitoes were responsible for the yellow fever outbreaks. Since 1881, Cuban physician Carlos Finlay had postulated that mosquitoes served as an intermediate host transmitting yellow fever to humans, but he had never proven his hypothesis because of miscalculations about the timing of yellow fever infectivity.[9] The case for mosquitoes as the culprit became stronger when, in 1898–1899, Italians Giovanni Grassi and Amico Bignami and English medical officer Ronald Ross demonstrated that anopheline mosquitoes spread malaria. In light of the suspicions about mosquitoes, Finlay provided Reed's commission with mosquito samples to start their own mosquito colony.[8]

Reed's commission first searched for evidence of a yellow fever bacterium in patients' blood. The group performed autopsies on 11 yellow fever victims but found no evidence of a bacterial yellow fever agent. The team's next step was more extreme. Two of the commission's researchers, Jesse Lazear and James Carroll, performed experiments on themselves. In August 1900, Lazear put an infected mosquito on Carroll's arm. After the bite, Carroll underwent a nearly deadly bout of yellow fever. Lazear became infected in September 1900, though it's unclear whether this infection was deliberate or accidental. Lazear was not as lucky as Carroll: he died of yellow fever on September 25, 1900.[8]

In additional experiments, American military personnel and Spanish immigrants volunteered to be (1) bitten by infected mosquitoes, (2) injected with the blood of yellow fever patients, or (3) isolated in rooms with materials covered in yellow fever's characteristic black vomit, urine, and feces.[8] Fortunately, Lazear would remain the only participant killed in the experiments. The Reed Commission concluded that *Aedes aegypti* was indeed the vector. The yellow fever virus spends 12 days in the mosquito before it can cause infections in humans. Bouts of yellow fever could also occur if a yellow fever patient's blood was injected into another person on the first or second day of the original patient's illness.[8]

The conclusive findings set off a crusade against mosquitoes in Havana in December 1900 that was overseen by William Gorgas, a career army doctor who had spent most of his professional life working in frontier medicine and administration in the American West. Dr. Gorgas designed a system with a distinctly military flavor to battle mosquitoes.[9] He divided Havana into sanitary districts that each had an assigned medical team. These teams maintained detailed file cards for every house and water source in their assigned districts. Based on this systematic data collection, brigades fanned across the Cuban capital to fumigate houses and drain, pour oil on, or cap various water sources, including wells, cisterns, and ponds. The strategy yielded impressive results. In just three months, the number of yellow fever cases plummeted from 1,400 to 37.[9] By the second half of 1901, Cuban health officials in Havana declared that there were no new cases of yellow fever in the capital.[8]

Militaristic Public Health beyond the Military: The Case of the Panama Canal

The US military's public health activities in Cuba and the Philippines also influenced the civilian sphere. The victory over yellow fever in Cuba occurred just as the United States was looking to make the dream of a canal through the Isthmus of Panama a reality. In the 1880s, the French attempt to construct a Central American canal was disastrous, and one of the most important causes of the failure was epidemic disease. An estimated 20,000 able-bodied workers died during the French construction project from mosquito-borne diseases, including yellow fever and malaria. Despite France's failure, the United States was eager to itself attempt to build a canal in Central America.[9] In her book chapter, "Yellow Fever Crusade: US Colonialism, Tropical Medicine, and the International Politics of Mosquito Control, 1900–1920," Alexandra Minna Stern chronicles the public health implications of US activities in the Canal Zone.[9]

The United States had deep economic and military interests in a Central American canal. The new, faster route between oceans would allow the country to ship economic goods more quickly and also enable faster movement of troops and weapons when at war. US diplomats saw these benefits and took action. In 1903, the United States used its growing clout to help Panama secede from Colombia through the Hay–Bunau-Varilla Treaty. As part of the treaty, the United States was given jurisdiction over a 50-mile by 10-mile "Canal Zone" in Panama, which it would retain for more than 90 years.[9]

The canal construction process employed about 60,000 West Indian, American, and European workers and lasted 10 years, from 1904 to 1914. Per Stern, the project was managed with meticulous detail by the Isthmian Canal Commission (ICC), which the United States formed to oversee the new possession. The ICC controlled almost every facet of workers' lives, including their work schedules, housing, food, and entertainment. The ICC's paternalistic role also extended to public health measures. Even outside the Canal Zone in the Panamanian cities of Panama City and Colón, the US Government was given the right to enter homes, remove standing water, and punish those who violated health codes. At one point during the canal's construction, all households in Panama City were ordered to get rid of gutters to eliminate standing water, and those who did not comply were fined or jailed. Panamanians who complained about intrusive measures were informed that they had no recourse since the United States had ultimate authority about health matters.[9]

It was in this environment that Dr. Gorgas was appointed chief sanitary officer for the canal project. Although there was still some skepticism about the role of mosquitoes in spreading disease, President Roosevelt pressured the ICC to give Gorgas the resources he needed for an aggressive sanitary campaign. With $50,000 in funding, Gorgas launched a relentless attack on the mosquitoes of the Canal Zone toward the end of 1905, replicating the approach from Cuba. Gorgas created 25 sanitary districts, each of which had an assigned inspector who led a team of 20 to 100 men. The brigades' activities included drainage projects; house inspections and fumigation; distribution of netting; spraying kerosene, sulfur, and alcohol to kill mosquitoes and their larvae; and digging ditches and water canals. In January 1906 alone, the teams inspected nearly 10,000 houses in Panama City, of which 1,785 had mosquito larvae. Gorgas's team made short work of yellow fever. By May 1906, Gorgas could already report complete yellow fever eradication in the Canal Zone.[9]

There was no doubt that the campaign against yellow fever in the Canal Zone was a resounding success, but the paternalistic approach had a mixed legacy. The militaristic focus on eliminating standing water and mosquitoes left most other diseases unaddressed. Upon its arrival in Panama in 1914, the Rockefeller Foundation found an astounding 80% hookworm infection rate in many parts of the country, and diseases like dysentery and pneumonia had similarly been left to fester. Rockefeller Foundation health officers working to reduce hookworm in Panama encountered increased suspicion and hostility from local communities who had recently endured the ICC's aggressive, intrusive sanitary measures. The Panamanian health system also remained anemic during and after the Canal's construction. The Rockefeller Foundation's International Health Board noted in its 1921 annual report, "The development of local initiative has been stifled by the paternalistic policy of the Canal Zone."[9]

The ICC health crusades at the Panama Canal were also highly racialized. As was so often the case in colonial health programs, making the tropics livable for White Americans and Europeans was the priority. Gorgas explained this in a 1913 speech at Johns Hopkins University's medical school, saying, "Our sanitary work at Panama will be remembered as the event which demonstrated to the white man that he could live in perfectly good health in the tropics; that from this period will be dated the beginning of the great white civilization in these regions."[9]

The focus on saving White lives led to calls for racial segregation in the Canal Zone. As White populations in the Canal Zone became healthier in the absence of disease-carrying mosquitoes, many began to attribute the White population's improved health to hygienic and "civilized" practices. In contrast, non-White workers and locals were perceived as a reservoir of disease because of "unhygienic" and "primitive" customs. The anti-mosquito measures added fuel to these racist interpretations of health in the Canal Zone. The ICC sanitary brigades spent considerably more time attacking mosquitoes in White workers' living quarters and did less to screen houses and eliminate standing water in the living quarters of non-White, West Indian laborers. This was deemed necessary because of the assumption that White workers were less immune to disease in the tropics.[9]

The disparity allowed disease rates to remain stubbornly high among non-White workers. The mortality rate from January to October 1906 was 59 per 1,000 among Black workers, almost four times as high as the 17 per 1,000 rate among White workers. In addition to the less robust anti-mosquito measures in non-White living quarters, the heightened mortality among non-White workers was also due to diseases like pneumonia and dysentery, which were overlooked by colonial medicine's heavy emphasis on yellow fever and malaria. The disregard for non-White workers' lives can still be seen in the mortality data that we have from the Canal Zone. Whereas mortality data for White employees include names, occupations, and ages, mortality data for Black workers is a simple tally.[9]

The US CDC's Military Roots

The military continued to strongly influence US global health later in the 20th century. In the United States today, most major federal agencies are based in or near Washington, DC. The Centers for Disease Control and Prevention (CDC) is an exception, with its headquarters in Atlanta, Georgia. The decision to place the CDC in Atlanta has its origins in military strategy during World War II. Yet the enemy that led to the creation of the CDC was neither Germany nor Japan. The CDC was created to battle a more ubiquitous foe: anopheline mosquitoes, the vector for malaria.

Historian Elizabeth Etheridge explores the CDC's military roots in depth in *Sentinel for Health: A History of the Centers for Disease Control*.[10] When the United States entered World War II in December 1941, malaria threatened American troops at training camps in the US South and fighting in the Pacific. In February 1942, Surgeon General Thomas Parran published a letter that established a new organization targeting malaria in the armed forces. Initially called the National Defense

Malaria Control Activities and then Malaria Control in Defense Areas, the organization was finally named Malaria Control in War Areas (MCWA) in April of the same year. Washington, DC, was too crowded with temporary federal offices to take on another government organization, so other locations were assessed. California and Texas were considered because of their relative proximity to the Pacific, but Georgia ultimately won because of its heavy malaria burden.[10]

MCWA was the earliest version of what became the CDC, and it could aptly be described as scrappy. The organization's first home was in a few rooms on the sixth floor of the Volunteer Building in downtown Atlanta. Most of the people with expertise on malaria were already working for the army, navy, and the PHS, so less than 10% of MCWA's commissioned officers had any prior experience in malaria control.[10]

In the spirit of efficiency and economy, MCWA's projects focused on larvicidal measures, primarily through pouring diesel oil on the still water where mosquitoes bred. The scope of the work was daunting. When MCWA was established in 1942, there were 900 "war establishments" to protect, including camps, bases, depots, shipyards, war factories, and housing for war workers. By the end of the war, the number of war establishments had ballooned to about 2,000. At that point, MCWA's purview had also expanded to include dengue and yellow fever, and DDT had become the weapon of choice against mosquitoes. DDT's devastating ecological impact wouldn't come to full light until Rachel Carson published *Silent Spring* in the 1960s. In the meantime, MCWA's anti-malaria campaign was considered a resounding success; malaria incidence was so low that there was talk of eradication.[10]

The success against malaria helped make the case for MCWA's survival. After the war, at the recommendation of Dr. Joseph Walter Mountin, MCWA leadership secured congressional approval for a more permanent organization. MCWA would live on with a new name starting in 1946: the Communicable Disease Center. Beyond the name, many other aspects of the organization were also poised to evolve.[10] In the aftermath of the war, anti-malaria efforts underwent a fundamental shift, largely thanks to the arrival of a new epidemiologist. In the late 1940s, Dr. Alexander Langmuir was an associate professor of epidemiology at Johns Hopkins University's School of Hygiene and Public Health. He surprised his colleagues when he left Johns Hopkins in 1949 to take charge of the Epidemiology Division at the CDC, which still was a relatively obscure agency.[10]

Langmuir arrived at the CDC when the DDT crusade against malaria was still in action, but he had a different vision for eradicating malaria. He imagined teams of four people in every state—including an epidemiologist, a nurse epidemiologist, an engineer, and an entomologist—with the epidemiologists investigating every case of malaria that was identified. If any cases were confirmed in laboratory tests, the engineer and entomologist would manage control measures in the surrounding area. The new model was approved on a small scale, and full-time malaria surveillance teams were dispatched to Mississippi and South Carolina, while part-time teams were sent to Georgia, Alabama, Arkansas, and Texas.[10]

But Langmuir included a crucial detail in his original memo about the new surveillance teams. He suggested that if there were no malaria cases to investigate, the team could investigate other kinds of epidemic disease. This ended up happening quickly: The first surveillance teams investigated leprosy in Louisiana and Florida, dysentery and polio in New Mexico, histoplasmosis in Kansas, and conjunctivitis in Georgia.[10]

The surveillance teams represented a paradigm shift in the meaning of "surveillance" in public health. Until the 1940s, surveillance referred to monitoring a person suspected of having a serious disease so that she or he could be isolated upon the first symptom. The year 1950 marked the first use of the term to describe monitoring of a disease instead of monitoring individual people. The new meaning reflected the systematic data collection and evaluation seen on Langmuir's surveillance teams.[10]

In the Cold War, Langmuir knew that the CDC had a role to play in the international standoff between the United States and the Soviet Union. In a 1949 meeting with state health officers, Langmuir warned that sabotage of food and water supplies would be the Soviets' and other enemies' first line of attack against the United States. He argued that epidemiology was the first line of defense since it could systematically track these types of attacks. That same year, the National Security Resources Board called on the nation to create a strategy against all manner of warfare, including bacteriological and chemical warfare. The outbreak of the Korean War in June 1950 gave even more energy and urgency to the calls for new strategies because of concerns about biological warfare.[10]

It was in this time of heightened anxiety about biological warfare that the Epidemic Intelligence Service (EIS) was born. In July 1950, Dr. Langmuir traveled to Washington, DC, for a Public Health Service meeting. The meeting focused on improving detection of covert biological warfare attacks. Attendees discussed how school and workplace absentee records could provide early clues to biological attacks. Langmuir emphasized the need for better epidemic reporting and routine case reporting. Over the next few hours, the meeting's attendees agreed to develop a stronger infrastructure for epidemiologic investigation.[10]

The day after the meeting in Washington, DC, the idea of "epidemiological intelligence" was approved at the Surgeon General's staff meeting. In the budgeting process that ensued, Langmuir proposed a core training team of six higher-level personnel. He also envisioned extensive investment in laboratory personnel and a recruitment strategy that would rely on the draft of doctors (which was already happening for the Korean War) and that would also look for medical school graduates with one or two years of medical experience.[10]

In July 1951, the first class of the EIS arrived for a six-week training in Atlanta, led by faculty from the Johns Hopkins School of Hygiene and Public Health. Of the 23 men in this first class, all but one were physicians. Their recruitment had been haphazard. Some had submitted applications, others responded to letters sent to medical and public health schools, and a few came from within the CDC itself. They underwent a very academic training, focused on Johns Hopkins's case-control study model, which would be emulated for years to come. At the end of the training, the students dispersed to different assignments in states, research universities, or CDC offices. Some EIS officers did malaria surveillance, which was the source of half the EIS budget. When the cohort gathered for the first EIS Conference in Atlanta in the spring of 1952, they each presented about their work for 10 minutes before fielding 10 minutes of questions.[10]

The EIS soon became known for rapidly answering calls for help against epidemics. In its first full year of existence, in 1952, EIS officers responded to more than 200 calls for assistance. Langmuir knew this on-call model to be effective and, perhaps just as importantly, exciting. He spoke of the work as "a hell of a lot more fun than dealing with the complexities of an academic situation. [We] throw them overboard. See if they can swim, and if they can't throw them a life ring, pull them out, and throw them in again."[10]

EIS's class size grew each year, and the CDC's reputation grew with it. The CDC director from 1983 to 1989, Dr. James Mason, emphasized the importance of Langmuir and EIS to the CDC's growth. He noted, "In the early days of CDC, it was really epidemiology, Langmuir, and the credibility of the EIS that brought a relatively small, obscure communicable disease center into the national light where it could grow and be appreciated. Instead of CDC becoming part of another organization, other organizations became a part of CDC."[10] Over the decades, EIS officers have made contributions to global health in areas as varied as smallpox eradication, poliovirus vaccine contamination, childhood lead poisoning, respiratory virus outbreaks, post-disaster response, and many other domains.[11]

Militaries in Contemporary Global Health

Positive and negative themes from earlier eras continue to define the military presence in global health. The main source of tension in military global health—which has echoed from colonial settings—is the commitment to advancing military objectives. Militaries' core mission is not to provide humanitarian aid or address public health issues. This primary commitment to defense can raise doubts about the effectiveness and intentions of military involvement in global health. Joshua Michaud et al. examine these tensions in their *Lancet* article, "Militaries and Global Health: Peace, Conflict, and Disaster Response."[12]

Skepticism about the military role in global health should not overshadow clear, positive achievements. Just as military personnel were heavily involved in research on yellow fever during the Spanish-American War in the late 19th century, militaries invest in cutting-edge global health research in the present day. As Michaud et al. note, US military researchers contributed to the development of the first approved malaria vaccine and the development of HIV vaccines that have entered Phase 3 vaccine trials. Chinese and US military personnel have also made contributions to Ebola vaccine and pharmaceutical research, and Australian military personnel have conducted research on dengue and malaria. The US Department of Defense is the fifth largest funder of neglected tropical disease research in the world.[12]

Militaries also contribute significantly to humanitarian responses in the wake of earthquakes, hurricanes, and other major disasters. In the aftermath of the 2010 earthquake in Haiti, 19 different militaries provided on-the-ground support. Militaries are often well-positioned to provide disaster-related aid because of their capacity for rapid mobilization on a large scale, in addition to budgets that often dwarf civilian disaster-response organizations. There are also examples of militaries helping to rebuild health systems in post-conflict contexts, as the Australian Defense Force did in both Rwanda and Timor-Leste.[12]

It is also common for militaries to build strategic health-training partnerships to strengthen allies' health-related capabilities, and perhaps even more importantly, build mutual goodwill. The US Department of Defense provided training and conducted exercises on pandemic preparedness and response in 16 African countries from 2008 to 2019, for example. Several militaries send out "hospital ships" for medical diplomacy missions in other countries, and China has sent medical units to African countries to build capacity for malaria and HIV/AIDS treatment.[12]

Despite these positive contributions, there is reason to be wary of military involvement in global health initiatives. Just as colonial-era global health focused on protecting soldiers and colonists, military global health research focuses primarily on acute infectious diseases that affect young adults (the demographic in military service) and on diseases that pose health security threats, such as anthrax and small-pox. Diseases impacting other populations, such as children, are less likely to attract military research.[12]

Another echo of the colonial era is the continued use of healthcare as a tool for winning over foreign civilian populations. The United States has made no secret of its attempts to "win the hearts and minds" of Vietnamese, Afghani, and Iraqi civilians through medical care provision and public health initiatives.[12] By generating more positive responses from civilian populations, the US military hoped to reduce attacks against American soldiers and gain more intelligence from local communities.[13] The United States is far from alone in using this tactic. In addition to other countries' militaries using healthcare as a strategic tool, non-state armed groups such as Sri Lanka's Tamil Tigers, Afghanistan's Taliban, and Lebanon's Hezbollah have all sought to win greater legitimacy by incorporating healthcare into their strategies.[12]

The positive role of militaries in global health is also counterbalanced by violations of the Geneva Conventions. The failure of armed forces to uphold the Geneva Conventions has led to infectious disease outbreaks in places including Syria and Yemen. More appalling is the deliberate targeting of healthcare workers and healthcare facilities; the Safeguarding Health in Conflict Coalition estimated that more than 700 attacks occurred on healthcare facilities and healthcare workers across 23 countries in 2017 alone.[12]

There is also a disconnect between militaristic, short-term approaches to global health and the long-term approaches that are needed to create lasting change. Militaries will often favor a solution that meets short-term objectives, such as deploying a humanitarian hospital ship.[12] And, of course, if military public health interventions are imposed without buy-in or understanding of local communities, interventions can do more harm than good. The overreaches of the US military a hundred years ago in Panama and the Philippines are all too easily replicated when viewing public health through a military lens.

Michaud et al. highlight the 2014–2015 West Africa Ebola epidemic as an example of contemporary military involvement in global health and its mixed record.[12] Militaries from the affected countries, Canada, China, Germany, France, the United Kingdom, the United States, and member states of the African Union made a wide range of contributions in transport, logistics, healthcare worker training, laboratory services, medical care, construction, burials, quarantine enforcement, and security.[12] Militaries were praised for rapid deployment of assets, well-trained professional staff accustomed to working in challenging environments, well-organized chains of command, strong communication, high-quality medical care provision, and boosting morale in the affected countries. Simultaneously, military involvement presented challenges. Foreign military deployments in West Africa were highly costly. The response was sometimes hindered by inflexible military policies, including some prohibitions against military providers offering direct patient care, certain rules against transporting laboratory samples, and insistence on adhering to non-local building codes for Ebola treatment units. Local military forces were also accused of employing unnecessary violence during the Ebola response, especially when enforcing quarantine. This violence eroded public trust in the overall response.[12]

The Rise of "Global Health Security"

Today, the notion of connecting global health and defense extends far beyond a purely military sphere. "Global health security" has become a buzzword in public health circles. The linking of health to "security" recognizes that public health issues (or "threats") can indeed be security issues, especially in the case of acute infectious disease outbreaks. In the last decade, the Global Health Security Agenda (GHSA) has emerged as the most formal international recognition of infectious disease outbreaks as security threats. GHSA arose after a string of alarming international outbreaks, including severe acute respiratory syndrome (SARS) in 2003, the H1N1 (swine flu) pandemic in 2009, West Africa's Ebola epidemic from 2014 to 2016, and outbreaks of cholera, chikungunya, Zika, and yellow fever over the same period. The outbreaks demonstrated the world's insufficient preparedness for infectious disease threats. Given that clear global vulnerability, 29 countries, the World Health Organization, the Food and Agriculture Organization of the United Nations, and the World Organization for Animal Health launched the GHSA in 2014.[14]

A critical characteristic of contemporary global health security is its focus on long-term capacity building. Today, GHSA includes 70 countries in addition to private sector companies and international and nongovernmental organizations. GHSA members come together to bolster the capacity to prevent, detect, and respond to infectious diseases on a national and international scale. By 2024, GHSA aims to have more than 100 countries complete an evaluation of their health security capacity and carry out identifiable improvements across multiple technical areas, including laboratory systems, surveillance, workforce development, and immunization.[15] Beyond GHSA, global health security initiatives generally focus on capacity building. Military interventions in global health have frequently faced criticism for favoring short-term solutions; global health security ideally addresses that issue by strengthening public health infrastructure over the long term.

Taking Stock of Militaries in Global Health

Early military involvement in global health was defined by colonialism. Navies that reinforced colonial empires were the initial bastions of "tropical medicine," and imperial rivalry fueled military health spending. Military involvement in global health could be well-organized and effective in stamping out disease but often alienated local populations through aggressive public health campaigns. Today, many global health institutions can still trace their roots to militaries. Contemporary military involvement in global health remains an opportunity and a challenge, with both positive impacts on health outcomes and questions about the appropriateness of militaries as global health actors.

Concluding Thoughts

BILL FOEGE

Just as colonialism may have been the most important negative influence on global health, unbelievably, for many, military medicine may have been the greatest positive influence on global health. From a marine perspective, and the creation of marine hospitals around the world, an interest in diseases of the tropics eventually led to schools of tropical medicine in many countries. This movement would expand from true tropical diseases to health problems in tropical countries, such as malnutrition, measles, pneumonia, and maternal mortality. This interest would lead to the current concept of global health, inclusive in a way that international health could never be.

In this country, military medicine and the marine hospitals produced the National Institutes of Health, the office of the Surgeon General, the CDC, the first medical teaching programs in this country, the VA hospital system, and even the US Public Health Service. The tragedy of war is heart-rending, but the contributions of military medicine deserve our gratitude.

But we dare not miss the delicate balance. While military medicine has led to the CDC and the Epidemic Intelligence Service, with uniformed Public Health Service officers being prepared to identify and respond to biological warfare, public health workers need to be under the direction of civilian authorities. Any concern that public health work is a cover for military or CIA intelligence gathering can only lead to trouble. On one occasion, as I worked on relief activities near the front lines during the Nigerian war, the CIA asked my supervisor, Dr. David Sencer, for permission to interview me. Dr. Sencer refused, saying our public health activities needed to avoid any implication that we were involved in the military or intelligence activities.

CHAPTER 5

Religious Missions and Global Health

MADISON GABRIELLA LEE

W hat inspired faith traditions and followers of those faiths to leave home, travel thousands of miles to another culture, often live in difficult conditions, and work for low salaries—all to share medical skills and knowledge?

From the beginning, reasons varied. For some, it was, indeed, an expression of faith or, relatedly, an urge to convert others to one's faith tradition. For some, it was a search for adventure. For still others, it was an attempt to escape their current situation.

Often medical expertise was requested to keep missionaries alive, rather than to benefit local populations. Not until later did medical staff share their skills with local citizens, and thereafter, mission programs found that medical programs were often the greatest attraction to local populations. It was a short step to use the medical programs to proselytize. It seemed so reasonable that it was often accepted without discussion. However, then the process became competitive, and in some areas, faith groups established medical facilities to compete with established programs run by other faith groups.

Colonial powers quickly saw the value of these medical programs and would frequently assist faith groups in establishing educational and medical facilities. These efforts helped colonial powers instill local populations with European economic and governmental ideals and religious and spiritual traditions.

Approaches also differed by geographic area. In this chapter, we contrast two adjacent countries' programs, focus on medical missions in three areas of the world, and, finally, discuss some specific problems, such as leprosy.

Dr. Albert Schweitzer in Gabon versus Missions in Present-Day Democratic Republic of the Congo

Albert Schweitzer was originally from Alsace, in the German Empire. He studied music and theology and had earned doctoral degrees in religion, philosophy, and music before the age of 30. He had a bright future in several fields had he stayed in Europe.

However, at age 30, he entered medical school and earned a fourth doctoral degree, this in medicine. Upon graduation, in 1912, he served in the village of Lambaréné in present-day Gabon, supported by the Paris Missionary Society.[1] He spent over half a century running a medical program there.

Early in his mission work, Dr. Schweitzer established a hospital in Lambaréné with his wife, Helene Bresslau. Work was interrupted during World War I, when the Schweitzers were placed in an internment camp and their hospital was destroyed. In 1924, Dr. Schweitzer and his assistant reestablished the hospital, which continued to evolve over the decades. Volunteer medical workers began to visit and assist. In the 1980s, a research laboratory was added, at the request of the Gabonese government, to focus on infectious diseases, including malaria and schistosomiasis.[2] Today, the hospital receives 50,000 patients annually.[3] The hospital long reflected French colonization and paternalism. However, in 2012, the hospital finally elected its first Gabonese director, Antoine Nziengui.[4]

At the outset, Dr. Schweitzer set out to "atone for the sins white Europeans had committed."[4] Dr. Schweitzer used medical missions and his practice to share his religious message by example.

However, in stark contrast were missionaries in the Congo Free State (1885–1907) and Belgian Congo (1908–1960). Although Protestant missionaries from the British Baptist Missionary Society (BMS) arrived before King Leopold II of Belgium acquired and took control of the Congo Free State, the king saw the missionaries as allies and encouraged their efforts. He also encouraged the missions of Belgian Catholics to the Congo.

Through contracts and funding, Catholic and Protestant missionaries and the colonial government were inextricably linked. Medical mission work, "whether carried on by qualified or unqualified staff . . . proved itself an indispensable branch of missionary service."[5] The missionaries often used medicine as an incentive for patients to accept their religious beliefs.

Despite the financial support and encouragement from King Leopold II, the missionaries were not properly equipped, even to care for their own expatriate community. Between 1878 and 1888, BMS reported that 50% of its missionaries died. From 1888 to 1898, around 33% of the missionaries died, and from 1898 to 1907, 21% of the missionaries died.[5]

Due to its original intent to promote the health and well-being of colonizers and fellow missionaries, the Congolese community, especially nonbelievers, were barred from receiving medical treatment. It was not until later that the medical missionaries used religious conversion as an entrance requirement to the hospital or medical practice. By the 20th century, however, the role of medical missionaries continued to evolve, with services eventually extended to the local community, whether converted or not.

Catholic missionaries also supported the education of the Congolese.[6] Education and schools were seen as large drivers of conversion. Yet the benefits of hospitals and schools cannot neutralize the fact that under Leopold II's colonial government, the Congolese population was exploited and forced into slavery for the extraction of rubber. According to *Low Countries Historical Review*:

Protestant missionaries were some of the earliest and most vocal in demanding an international accounting for the atrocities being committed under this system. The Catholic orders were largely silent, a troubling passivity.[7]

Indeed, a number of priests became active participants in the slave trade.

Faith-Based Medical Programs in Africa, China, and India

Faith-based medical programs became widespread throughout the world, including in the United States, all of Africa, Central and South America, and Southeast Asia. Such programs also extended to China and Japan.[8] (Christian missionaries were prohibited in Japan until 1858, when the United States and Japan signed the Treaty of Amity and Commerce, and they were prohibited from much of China until 1860, when the Second Opium War ended.)

Africa

While Dr. Schweitzer, as discussed previously, set out to right the wrongs of other Europeans, other medical missionaries sometimes termed their time as "civilizing missions," but, ironically, the participants often could not even be civilized in dealing with each other. In the Congo Free State, Catholic and Protestant missionaries were frequently at odds throughout the 19th century. It would not be until the latter part of that century that the idea of unity among Christian denominations was seriously discussed.

David Livingstone was a Protestant missionary funded by the London Missionary Society. He documented many of his observations throughout southern Africa; they primarily described the influence of the Jesuits (Catholic missionaries). He noted their success in increasing literacy but failure in maintaining religious practices. For Livingstone, the "civilizing mission" meant Christianity and commerce. However, he did not agree with the Jesuits' introduction of commerce through the slave trade.[9]

Livingstone also believed that healthcare and mission service should go hand in hand. While colonizers and missionaries were trying to keep one another alive, they established numerous hospitals. As described for the missions in the present-day Democratic Republic of Congo, eventually access to those hospitals was not restricted solely to colonizers and/or missionaries.

Many mission hospitals exist to this day; however, in some sub-Saharan African countries, governments have taken over ownership. In 2007, the African Religious Health Assets Programme produced a report on Lesotho and Zambia for the World Health Organization (WHO). In Lesotho, approximately 40% of national health services were estimated to be provided by 9 Christian hospitals and 75 health centers, whose managing churches are members of the Christian Health Association of Lesotho. In Zambia, the numbers were similar, with 30% of services provided by 30 hospitals and 66 rural health centers, whose managing churches are members of the Churches Health Association of Zambia.[10] Even excluding the medical facilities taken over by governments in the last 60 years, an analysis in 2012 reported that approximately 6.8% of inpatient and outpatient healthcare in sub-Saharan Africa was still being provided by faith-based organizations.[11]

The early bias of some medical missions against local populations had other ramifications. In the late 20th century, the Tanzania Muslim Professionals Organization and Muslim Solidarity Trust Fund "aimed at curtailing the alleged marginalization of Muslims in the country, which, they argue, has become most palpable in the fields of health and education."[12] Muslim revivalists believe that the entanglement between the government, international donors, and missionaries made Tanzania a "Christian state." Today, Christian and Muslim organizations are still competing for territory through medical missions. Their missions have dual motivations—one addressing health and social inequality and the second exerting political and social impact.

Ophthalmology in China

As early as 2600 BC and into the 19th century, Chinese practitioners relied on pulse diagnoses.[13,14] In that practice, over a dozen pulses were used to assess each of the internal organs. The pulse rate was based on the ratio between pulse and respiration; a normal pulse rate was four beats to one respiration.[15] An irregular pulse rate was believed to be caused by the imbalance of yin and yang—two interrelated forces.[13] Additionally, Chinese practitioners treated ailments; diseases were treated with acupuncture, herbs, and powders.

Surgeries, especially those of the eye, were not performed. This created a unique opportunity for medical missionaries to use their knowledge of surgeries, and other Western medicine, to evangelize. However, given the relations between China and Western countries throughout the 19th century, foreigners were restricted to Canton and Macao. Dr. Robert Morrison, a Protestant minister, regarded as the "Father of China Mission" by some, spent over 25 years in Macao to compile the first Chinese-English dictionary and translate the Bible into Chinese.[14]

Between 1819 and 1834, the American Board of Commissioners for Foreign Missions (ABCFM) sent several doctors to China after some missionaries funded by the board had died. Among those doctors was Dr. Peter Parker, the first Protestant medical missionary to go to that country.

Parker earned a bachelor's degree, a medical degree, and a theological degree from Yale University in the 1830s. Waiting to start his mission, he supplemented his degree with one week at the eye infirmary and hospital in New York City. That one week later proved to be crucial to his work in China.

Parker arrived in Canton in 1834. He was initially sent with the intentions of spending minimal time on the medical work of the local community; instead, he was supposed to protect the health of three fellow American Board missionaries—Elijah Coleman Bridgman, S. Wells Williams, and Edwin Stevens.

However, with only three missionary patients, Parker decided to dedicate his energy and resources toward the community in Canton.

In 1835, one year after his arrival, he opened an ophthalmic infirmary in Canton. Parker chose this practice because diseases of the eyes were prevalent, and Chinese medicine had not yet used surgical therapies. The main surgical technique he used was couching, to treat cataracts. This technique required Parker to insert a needle through the cornea to push the cataract inside the eye. This technique requires a long recuperation time and makes the eye vulnerable to other ailments; however, the procedure was deemed to be relatively simple. "Within the first four months of his Canton practice he had couched some thirty cataracts with only two failures."[14] It was said that Parker "opened China to the gospel at the point of a lancet."[16]

In addition to cataracts, there is evidence that trachoma was also a widespread issue. Even though the bacterium causing trachoma, *Chlamydia trachomatis*, was not discovered until the 1970s, historical accounts (including Parker's) suggest its presence. He described patients with "chronic ophthalmia," "granulations of the lid," and "pannus." One of his entries described treating the patient with

> sixteen leeches applied to the temple, sulphate of copper to the granulations, collyrium of nitrate of silver used daily, calomel and rhubarb at night, syringing of the eyes, scarifying the lids, and once again applying sulphate of copper.[14]

After several months of this treatment, the patient had completely recovered. Washes of copper sulphate were used throughout the 20th century for trachoma, but today it is treated with trichiasis surgery and an oral antibiotic, azithromycin.[14,17]

However, this was not the only procedure Parker was conducting. While his infirmary was intended to focus on ophthalmology, he treated other ailments and diseases, and performed hysterectomies and mastectomies.

By establishing his hospital, Dr. Parker not only created a new type of mission enterprise in China, which became a staple among mission institutions; he also opened new kinds of relationships with the Chinese.[14] The infirmary was met with skepticism because there were no fees for the services, and Parker was placed under official surveillance.

However, despite that initial distrust, 925 patients were seen at the infirmary within the first quarter.

When given the chance with these patients, Dr. Parker evangelized. His approach to medical missions was to "liberate man from physical, mental, and moral vassalage, and to disseminate the blessings of science and Christianity all over the globe."[14]

Parker went on to open a second hospital, in Macao, in 1838. That same year, he established the Medical Missionary Society of China with Thomas College, an English surgeon.[18] Both hospitals and the Medical Missionary Society were hindered by the First Opium War (1839–1842); however, patients still visited Parker until his departure in 1840. In 1842, he returned with his wife, Harriet, and reopened the hospital in Canton.

Even though Parker continued his work at the hospital in that site, the ABCFM terminated its sponsorship. The American Board believed his diplomatic affairs and medical work outweighed his evangelistic work.[16]

This was a recurring theme in medical missions. Many saw medical work as a mechanism for proselytizing, rather than an end in itself. Failure to get converts could end the medical investment. Parker worked at the hospital until returning to the United States in 1855.

Later, in 1861, Parker's fellow missionary, Dr. William Lockhart, founded another hospital in Peking—the foundation for the Peking Union Medical College. In 1915, the Rockefeller Foundation purchased the medical college from the London Missionary Society. The year before, the foundation had established the China Medical Board.

Maternal and Child Health in India

At the inception of medical missions, women were often told that "their principal and usually only duty was to render their home a heaven, and their husband happy by lightening his cares, training his children, soothing his sorrows, sympathizing in his stresses, and lending their counsel and support to his duties."[19] However, when the missionary community noted that its gospel message was not reaching women, an opportunity opened up for women; the missionary community recognized that it needed to send educated women on missions. The Women's Union Missionary Society of America for Heathen Lands, a nondenominational organization, was established in 1861 specifically to send single women into the mission field.

Two decades later, in 1881, a report by the Presbyterian Board garnered further support for sending single women into the mission field. The Presbyterian Board recognized that, given the cultural and religious norms of certain communities, male physicians lacked access to women in need of medical assistance.[19] By 1893, the Women's Union had sent 65 women to China, India, and Japan; other American and European missionary boards had also sponsored single-women missionaries. That year, women represented approximately 60% of active missionaries in these areas.[19]

And women continued to advocate for their right to serve in foreign missions. Mrs. D. W. Thomas was one of those advocates. As a Methodist missionary wife in North India, she wrote to the Women's Union Missionary Society, asking for women medical missionaries to train girls at her orphanage in medical work.[20,21] Dr. Clara Swain and Isabella Thoburn were the earliest single-women missionaries to be sponsored by a women's foreign missionary society from North America. Correspondence between Thoburn and her brother revealed that he questioned women's ability to contribute to the field, even his sister's. Not until later was it noted that "a Christian woman sent out to the field was a Christian missionary, and that her time was as precious, her work as important, and her rights as sacred as those of the more conventional missionaries of the other sex."[19] Thoburn was a champion of equal access to education and went on to contribute to the higher education of women in India, including the founding of Thoburn College and assisting and training other local teachers. Dr. Swain went on to set up the earliest women's hospitals in India.

As the careers of Swain and Thoburn illustrate, this new opportunity for women meant that they could contribute to the advancement of women's education, health, and spiritual well-being in the communities to which they were sent. In the early 20th century, Dr. Ida Scudder was a prominent advocate for maternal and child health. Members of her large family were American missionaries in India, including her father, physician Dr. John Scudder. In a single night, three local men needing medical assistance for their pregnant wives visited the Scudder family. Even though Dr. Scudder was present, each of the men only wanted Ida's assistance. Knowing that she could not help—because she was not medically trained—Ida did not follow any of the men to help their wives. The following day, she learned that all three women had died in childbirth; as a result, she was spurred to study medicine.

After doing so, in America, the now-Dr. Ida Scudder returned to India. Though first met with skepticism, she became known for her "roadside" clinics among rural patients. With the support of the Reformed Church in America, she opened the Mary Taber Schell Memorial Hospital, and with interdenominational cooperation, she founded one of the most prestigious women's medical colleges in the country, the Christian Medical College Vellore.[20,22] At the medical college, Dr. Scudder delivered many messages that "meshed medical service and professionalism with issues of gender, health, and social responsibility."[20]

Even before the Vellore school opened, the Ludhiana Christian Medical College was started, in 1894, to train women as doctors. Dame Edith Mary Brown, an English doctor, not only started the medical college but also served as principal for half a century. It is an outstanding medical school to this day. Yet its beginnings broke the norm: most medical schools started with male students, later admitting females. Brown, Scudder, and Swain started training programs for females, and only later allowed men to be trained there.

Like Drs. Scudder and Brown, others perceived the need to address maternal and child health. Dr. Anna Dengel, an Austrian physician, served as a mission doctor for four years in India. She witnessed women die in childbirth who had refused care from male physicians, due to cultural and religious restrictions. Her efforts to diagnose and treat diseases, in addition to her lack of social support, led to both mental and physical exhaustion—but also to her hope for a community of sisters working alongside her in the medical mission field:

I was fire and flame. . . . This was the answer to my subconscious desires and aspirations, to be a Missionary with a definite goal in view, filling an un-fulfilled need which only women could fill.[23]

More specifically, Dr. Dengel saw the need for a change in Roman Catholic legislation. At the time, Roman Catholics prohibited women from professional work, including obstetrics and surgeries. At the most, women were able to stand behind a curtain and hand the doctor instruments during a surgery.[23] Throughout the 1930s and 1940s, Dengel continuously expressed her thoughts on the interplay between religion and science in her journal, *Medical Missionary*.[23]

After successfully lobbying for changes to the Catholic Canon Law that forbade Catholic sisters from aiding in childbirth, Dengel established the first Roman Catholic congregation of women in 1941, called the Medical Mission Sisters.[23,24] This Catholic community continued to address the needs of women and the influence of their mission work through the Second Vatican Council (1962–1965).[23] The Second Vatican Council encouraged missionaries to engage with the local community, including shamans and traditional midwives.

The Medical Mission Sisters are cited as training Indian medical personnel and nurses, in addition to advocating for governments to provide adequate healthcare. Dengel and the Medical Mission Sisters also acknowledged the value in learning about the local culture, religious practices, and social norms to determine how each affected the health of women; in short, these women acknowledged social determinants of health:

> The roots of the conditions we have just examined lie far deeper than a mere lack of medical care. They are grounded in the social and economic indigence of missions . . . all over the world. All endeavor can avail but little unless it is accompanied throughout by a great effort, a striving toward the realization of a Christian ideal in our basic social and economic structure.[23]

In contrast to earlier missionaries, particularly those during the colonial era, Dengel ensured that the Medical Mission Sisters were not using baptism or conversion as requirements for medical care; the sisters were to care for all individuals, regardless of religious beliefs or customs. She noted that they were responding to what we "owe to the peoples subjected and exploited by our Forefathers."[25] By 1980, the Medical Mission Sisters had 700 members from 18 different countries working in 34 countries, including India.[24]

Both Drs. Scudder and Dengel used religious medical missions as means to advance maternal and child health and empower women to pursue healthcare.

Leprosy in India

Skin diseases were described in texts in India as early as 2000 BC. These diseases have since been determined to be leprosy, or Hansen's disease. This disease affects nerves, which leads to the inflammation and redness of the skin. Even as early as 2000 BC, individuals suspected to have leprosy were ostracized from society. "Ancient Indian society marginalized those with leprosy because of several factors: its chronic, potentially disfiguring nature; inconsistently effective therapy; association with sin; and the fear of contagion."[26]

Leprosy persisted throughout the colonialization of India and was influential in the direction of the missionary field. For some Christian missionaries, helping lepers was exactly what the Bible prescribed, and they were imitating the actions of Jesus in the New Testament.

> The evangelization of the world depends on the indigenous people of each nation, and what better missionary could be found than the leper cured of his disease, going back to his people telling them out of the fullness of his heart, the twofold gospel of spiritual and physical healing.[27]

Governments, like much of society, tended to avoid contact with lepers. So, church groups became a dominant force in providing care. Leprosy was endemic in Africa and Asia but rare in Europe. In 1872, the colonial government conducted a census and found 108,000 cases throughout the Indian population. By 1874, Norwegian physician

Gerhard Armauer Hansen identified the bacterium causing leprosy, *Mycobacterium leprae*. In his honor, the disease is often called Hansen's disease.[26] In 1889, Belgian missionary priest Father Damien died after contracting leprosy. He had served Hawaiian lepers for nearly three decades; his death brought increased attention to the plight of those with the disease.[28]

Colonists and missionaries both believed that lepers needed to be isolated. A missionary, Wellesley Cosby Bailey, visited the asylums housing the isolated lepers. This visit encouraged him to help the mental, physical, and spiritual conditions of India's lepers by founding the Mission to Lepers.[8]

Even with these asylums, colonial powers continued to experience pressure to address lepers. The colonial government enacted the Lepers Act of 1898, which required medical and social segregation of those afflicted with leprosy. Out of 200 million individuals in the 1890s, an estimated 250,000 were afflicted with the disease. The colonial government recognized that to place 250,000 individuals in isolation would be costly. Such costs provided an opening for mission societies. The government passed on the cost to mission societies, and in turn, provided them with authority and protection to evangelize.[8] The government did not, however, pass the entire cost to mission societies; they provided monthly stipends to fund leper asylums. By 1910, approximately 4,500 European missionaries from 130 missionary societies served in India.[8]

Secular organizations and societies were also commissioned to help with leprosy. In 1923, Leonard Rogers established the British Empire Leprosy Relief Association (BELRA) to help control leprosy.

Robert Greenhill Cochrane was an influential medical missionary with both Mission to Lepers and BELRA; however, his résumé as a leprologist extends well beyond the two societies. Cochrane was born in Pei-Tei-Ho, China, to missionary parents right before the Boxer Rebellion. In 1924, he served with the Mission to Lepers (The Leprosy Mission, present-day). He published a definitive textbook on leprosy and retired to the London School of Tropical Medicine.

One of us (Bill Foege) spent three days at Cochrane's home in 1965 before going to Africa. Cochrane's reasoning was that he could not live with his conscience if he allowed Foege to go to Africa knowing as little about leprosy as he seemed to know! Cochrane was the first to use the parent sulfone dapsone, or DDS, to treat leprosy. Today, multidrug therapy is the standard, including the use of dapsone with clofazimine and rifampicin.

Dr. Paul Brand was also influential in addressing leprosy in India. Cochrane and Brand both worked in the Christian Medical College Vellore. Brand pioneered reconstructive surgery that helped restore the mobility of the "clawed hand" that afflicts lepers.[29]

A Major Change in Medical Missions

One of the great revolutions in medical missions occurred in the 1960s and 1970s. The World Council of Churches established the Christian Medical Commission (CMC) in 1968 as a semiautonomous body to assist the World Council of Churches in its evaluation of, and assistance with, church-related medical programs in the developing world.

The decision to create the CMC evolved from much fieldwork and a series of consultations. The fieldwork, which started in late 1963, showed that churches had concentrated on hospital and curative services and that these "had a limited impact" in meeting the health needs of the people they were meant to be serving. It was found that "95% of church-related work was curative" and "at least half of the hospital admissions were for preventable conditions"![30]

According to reports from the CMC, the theological basis for health and healing work continued as important points of discussion during its first annual meetings. These were critical in helping the commission advise the World Council of Churches on how to help church-funded services move from the provision of medical care to individuals to the development of curative and preventive services to communities at large.

The discussions took the form of a dialog between Dr. John H. Bryant, the commission's chairman and a professor of public health, and David E. Jenkins, a commission member and theologian. The last dialog, which took place in 1973, demonstrates to what degree—even though there were important differences of opinion between the two—both men were committed to a distribution of resources that improved the lot of the most disenfranchised. This constituted a marked departure from the early objective of using medicine to improve conversions. The debates were published in a series of reports in *Contact*, a newsletter from the CMC.

James C. McGilvray, a dynamic leader, was instrumental in implementing the commission findings with three important developments. McGilvray had been superintendent of the Vellore Medical College Hospital and had experience with medical mission programs. First, he advised missions to work directly with the newly created post-colonial governments. Second, he promoted the idea that various faith groups should work together. In some countries, this resulted in a single person representing all Protestant work, able to represent them in discussions with the government health ministry. In at least one African country, the Protestant leader and the Catholic leader shared an office. Third, he promoted the idea of faith groups developing community and prevention programs.

Concluding Thoughts
BILL FOEGE

I spoke at a retreat in Kenya on incorporating prevention and community approaches in the hospital and clinical work then being done. James McGilvray, the first director of the CMC, had organized the retreat as part of his effort to take the message of community medicine to medical missionaries.

One story bears repeating because it illustrates what a consummate force McGilvray was in getting a fractious community to work together. At the end of the first day, an Irish priest had a communion service and invited missionary health workers from many denominations. I was impressed with this gesture—one I had never witnessed before. At the end of the day, McGilvray invited the Catholic priest, me, and a third person up to his room. He pulled out four glasses and poured whiskey. When he gave a glass to the priest, McGilvray said as an aside, "I have another bottle in my suitcase." The priest said, "Oh good, you gave me such a fright."

It is also worth mentioning that, a few years later, I received a letter from a surgeon who had attended that meeting. He wrote that it had changed his life and that he had just received an MPH degree from Johns Hopkins.

CMC's impact was significant. But it also provided another leadership initiative of lasting influence. A new director-general of WHO, Dr. Halfdan Mahler of Denmark, having read the materials reported in *Contact*, advised WHO staff to read the February 1973 issue (no. 13) on rural health. Soon, a joint CMC/WHO working group had been formed, and many of the CMC proposals were discussed at the 1978 meeting in Alma-Ata, Soviet Union, sponsored by both WHO and the Soviet Government. CMC's impact on WHO was so profound that the ripple effects continue to this day.

The positive impact of medical missions is obvious in the institutions around the world that continue—even if the faith-based origins are obscured by current government or secular sponsorship. The work often was an expression of beliefs that saw all people as equally deserving of the gifts of medical science. Attention to persons with leprosy is an example of providing care to the most disenfranchised. Likewise, the introduction of eye surgery to China was a positive aid that can't be discounted. The attention to the health of women and the creation of medical schools for females in India are counterintuitive to the expectations of colonialism or commercial interests. The important and lasting influence on WHO is of special interest, and many global health workers today still spring from a faith-based orientation and philosophy.

But even with religious medical work, there was a price to be paid. The examples of local populations ignored in order to treat colonial or mission staff are depressing. The obligation to falsely state a religious belief as the price for getting treatment is obscene. Such practices corrupt both providers and patients. Faith-based medical work thus displays both contributions and disappointments, with a higher tragedy cost than is usually acknowledged.

CHAPTER 6

Early Academic Programs

DEBORAH CHEN TSENG

O n May 8, 1980, the World Health Organization (WHO) declared
that smallpox had been eradicated.[1] This disease killed over 300
million people in the 20th century alone and had haunted humans for
thousands of years.[1] Yet while many of us living in contemporary society know that smallpox was eradicated, the implications of this
achievement do not carry as much weight as they would have had we
lived in a time prior to smallpox eradication, when 3 out of every 10
infected people died.[2]

Smallpox is only one of two diseases that WHO has declared eradicated; the other is rinderpest, a lethal viral disease of cattle. Neither
achievement could have occurred without the foundations laid by early
university programs in public health and medicine.[3] This chapter focuses on the history and establishment of three different schools of
public health: the Johns Hopkins School of Hygiene and Public Health,
the London School of Hygiene & Tropical Medicine, and Tulane University's School of Hygiene and Tropical Medicine.

Johns Hopkins School of Hygiene and Public Health:
Established 1916

During the early months of the COVID-19 pandemic, many around
the world turned to the Johns Hopkins University Bloomberg School

of Public Health for the most up-to-date data on the spread of the disease. More than a century ago, Johns Hopkins was faced with the 1918 flu pandemic, as the school welcomed its first student class. This was an event many years in the making, culminating in the Rockefeller Foundation's award of $267,000 to Johns Hopkins to establish a school of public health in 1916.

The History

John D. Rockefeller, who earned his fortune from Standard Oil, saw public health as a means by which he could partake in "scientific philanthropy." This was a phrase promoted by Andrew Carnegie, an industrialist and philanthropist known for the Carnegie Steel Company, Carnegie Library, and Carnegie Institute of Science, among many other organizations. This philanthropy focused on supporting systematic social improvement—such as the creation of libraries—that many could benefit from, as opposed to charity, which might benefit just a few. Additionally, both Rockefeller and Carnegie were interested in science and health, public health, and medicine; however, the term *scientific philanthropy* may have promised more precision than was possible.

From 1909 to 1914, the Rockefeller Sanitary Commission for the Eradication of Hookworm Disease tried to eradicate hookworm in the American South. This commission, run by Frederick T. Gates, Charles Wardell Stiles, and Wickliffe Rose, served as Rockefeller's business, scientific, and philanthropic adviser. Its members believed that the economic "backwardness" of the American South, as well as the lack of industrialization compared to the American North, could be explained by anemia caused by hookworm. While the commission did not succeed in eradicating hookworm, it was successful in discovering how helpful and important public health could be. Its public health propaganda—promoting anthelmintic drugs, wearing shoes, and the use of latrines—reduced both the incidence and risk of hookworm infection. Perhaps more importantly, the commission became aware that no distinct education or career paths existed for those pursuing public health in the nation's many medical schools, nursing schools, and established hospitals.

Indeed, most public health officers were practicing doctors who had been pulled into the response whenever there was a crisis and left after the crisis had been addressed. Moreover, most public health officers at the time were political appointees and, as such, had an active interest in not going against local political interests that might endanger their appointment.[4] So, while public health practices were found to be successful in the fight against hookworm, the men and women who were brought in to run the programs had little dedication to public health or to continuing programs to address it. It was this realization that led the Executive Committee of the International Health Board of the Rockefeller Foundation to pass a resolution stating that "the General Education Board be requested to consider the desirability of improving medical education in the United States, with a special view to the training of men for public health service," on December 19, 1913.[4] This statement was then followed by the convening of a meeting of the Rockefeller Foundation's General Education Board to discuss what an education in public health might look like.

The conference, which took place on October 16, 1914, was led by Wickliffe Rose, one of Rockefeller's advisers, and Abraham Flexner. In 1910, Flexner had published the groundbreaking Flexner Report, which led to the creation of medical schools as we know them, established the biomedical model as the gold standard, and led to the elimination of proprietary and for-profit medical schools. So, Flexner was no stranger to the proposal of a new or different education system.

It was at this conference that Rose proposed the idea that public health education be associated with a research-focused, science-founded school that would be separate from any medical school. Graduates from such a system would be used to create a network of public health officials across the United States who could respond to any outbreaks that might occur. In addition to this central hub for public health education, this school would be linked to a network of sister state schools, whose graduates would work together to promote public health. These schools would offer short-course and extension courses to allow for opportunities to upgrade the skills of the health officers. And since these school were to be spread across the country, they would be more easily accessible for graduates than returning to their alma mater.

Decades earlier, the state of Massachusetts had instituted a variety of requirements regarding public health. In 1874, the Massachusetts State Board of Health instituted a voluntary plan for physicians to report the diseases that they saw weekly in their patients.[5] In 1884, the state passed legislation requiring the reporting of "diseases dangerous to the public" and even fined those who did not participate in these reports; in short, such reporting was no longer voluntary.[6] Finally, in 1907, Massachusetts passed a law that required the reporting of cases of 16 different diseases.[7] However, to make use of the data, people needed to be trained in public health. As the Centers for Disease Control and Prevention did not come into existence until 1946, this mandate purportedly predated *national* reporting.[8] (However, in 1878, Congress had authorized collecting morbidity reports by the Public Health Service to control the quarantinable diseases of cholera, smallpox, plague, and yellow fever. In 1925, all the states began to report regularly. The official mechanism for reporting all of these data eventually became CDC's *Morbidity and Mortality Weekly Report* [Mike Gregg, editor of *MMWR*, pers. comm., 1980].)

Perhaps in slight contrast to the idea of "scientific philanthropy," Rose's ideas homed in on the biomedical aspects of public health. His ideas, centered around research, paid little attention to policy or plans for social or economic reforms to address the root of these issues.

This conference and the many subsequent discussions that took place concerning structured public health professional education were summarized in what would be called the 1915 Welch-Rose Report. Submitted to the Rockefeller Foundation, it would become the template for professional public health education both in the United States and abroad.[9]

Using the Welch-Rose Report as a guide, Johns Hopkins University was chosen from four different institutions that competed for funding from the Rockefeller Foundation to establish the first public health institute in the United States, in 1916.[10] Beating out Columbia University, Harvard University, and the University of Pennsylvania, Johns Hopkins was chosen based on the potential the committee thought its medical school would provide. Indeed, according to the final report from the General Education Board, the authors wrote:

> [The medical school is] the University's greatest asset. . . . It is a genuine University department, on the clinical as well as the laboratory side. The faculty is a small body, and since the introduction of the full-time scheme, entirely homogenous in character, animated by high ideals and very efficiently led.[10]

The value that Rose, Flexner, and Jerome Greene—a prominent New York philanthropist—placed on the medical school is understandable, given the importance they placed on biomedical and research aspects of public health. However, it would be remiss to ignore the fact that Columbia, Harvard, and the University of Pennsylvania had superior departments in terms of resources (e.g., opportunities for fieldwork, experienced public health teachers and researchers, scientific talent), which could have supported the newly established public health institute. Harvard had many advantages that would have made it an excellent location for the Rockefeller Foundation investment. It had a progressive and cooperative health department in Boston with many opportunities for fieldwork and hands-on experience along with a talented and experienced faculty and staff in the field of public health. Columbia University also had an excellent public health nursing program as well as a progressive and cooperative health department in New York, much like Harvard.

By contrast, Hopkins had few facilities that could be used to study infectious diseases, a health department that was not as progressive and cooperative as Boston or New York, and fewer faculty who were fully dedicated to public health. However, all of these factors were ignored in light of its medical school, which, while it had a small faculty, was "animated by high ideals and efficiently led."[4]

The final report *did* acknowledge these facts, noting that "the general resources of the University and the community are inferior—in some respects much inferior—to those found in New York, Boston and Philadelphia."[10] However, Rose, Flexner, and Greene placed the value of a medical school far above these social and, potentially, economic aspects.

This appraisal is perhaps unsurprising. It falls in line with the pre-established pattern of how the Rockefeller Sanitary Commission for the Eradication of Hookworm Disease tried to eradicate hookworm from the American South: the commission ignored the social and economic factors that influenced the prevalence and spread of hookworm. Additionally, Rose highly valued the biomedical aspect of public health and thought that whatever school was established would focus heavily on research.

That said, there is more to this story than what is traditionally told. What most historical accounts ignore is the fact that Welch, who had a hand in writing the Welch-Rose Report, was a professor of pathology at Johns Hopkins Medical School. Furthermore, he was the one to meet Rose, Flexner, and Greene during their visit to Johns Hopkins and to answer all of their questions concerning barriers and facilitators to the creation of an institute of public health at Johns Hopkins. Having written the report, one cannot deny that he knew exactly what they were looking for in a school and location. Additionally, there is plausible reason to believe, when reading the transcripts and questions from the committee's visit to Hopkins, that work done behind the scenes painted Hopkins in the best light possible.[4]

Abraham Flexner was most certainly biased toward Johns Hopkins, given his long-term friendship with and admiration for Welch.[4] Given this relationship, Flexner would have certainly known of Welch's desire for an institute of public health. In fact, in Flexner's own autobiography, he wrote:

> Someone in each of these centers had more or less vague ideas,
> but one man alone possessed the requisite knowledge and vision.
> I reported to Rose that it was immaterial where the school was
> located; it mattered only who directed it. The only possible director,
> in my opinion, was Dr. Welch; the school might be placed wherever
> he wished (p. 51).[4]

Welch became the first dean of the Johns Hopkins School of Hygiene and Public Health. Flexner's desires were achieved, as well as Welch's.

While Flexner was set on Hopkins, Greene was actually most impressed by Harvard.[4] However, after the committee decided on Hopkins and the Rockefeller Foundation provided it with the endowment, Greene's relationship with Harvard soured due to former president Charles W. Eliot's correspondence and fury over the decision.[4] He argued with Flexner that the only reason the committee decided on Hopkins was due to Welch. Based on transcripts, questions, and reports, Eliot may not have been wrong. Receiving little sympathy from Flexner, Eliot turned to Greene to air his concerns. However, Greene strongly rebuked him saying that "the attitude of the President [of Harvard] and the Corporation has made it difficult, if not impossible, for me to have any further relations of an official nature with the University."[4] Thus, Rose was the deciding vote when it came to choosing the location for the institute of public health, and he chose Baltimore and Hopkins.

In the end, Johns Hopkins received $267,000 to establish an institute of public health. The Johns Hopkins School of Hygiene and Public Health was born.

The Impact of Johns Hopkins School of Hygiene and Public Health

In 1913, E. V. McCollum, who would go on to be the new school's founding professor and chair of biochemistry (or, as it was then known, chemical hygiene), published a paper noting how certain lipids were needed in the diet of rats to promote growth.[11] These lipids were, in fact, vitamins A and D.[12] It was later found that xerophthalmia, or night blindness, as well as failure to thrive were associated with vitamin A deficiency in children, and rickets was associated with a lack of vitamin D.

Dr. Alfred Sommer, a professor at Johns Hopkins School of Hygiene and Public Health and later dean from 1990 to 2005, built on these early reports. His research found that even a mild vitamin A deficiency in children dramatically increased their risk of death from infectious diseases. Studies later found that, annually, more than a million children died and half a million children went blind due to vitamin A deficiency. Controlled trials conducted by Dr. Sommer discovered that 2 cents worth of vitamin A taken orally twice a year could prevent both deaths and blindness, a major advance for global health.[13] UNICEF and other agencies used these findings to support vitamin A supplementation and fortification. These programs are now in place in more than 70 low- and middle-income countries around the world.[13] The impact that this finding from Johns Hopkins has had on the lives of millions of children and their families is unquantifiable but helps to show the importance of public health and global health.

The US Public Health Service seconded Dr. Wade Hampton Frost to begin the first department of epidemiology. He had wide field experience and made epidemiology an academic subject that is now the basic science behind all of public health. He later became dean of the school.[13]

In the 1940s, a Johns Hopkins School of Hygiene and Public Health polio research team comprised of David Bodian, Howard Howe, and Isabel Morgan proved that poliovirus was transmitted orally, rather than via inhalation, as was previously thought. Their research also showed that paralytic polio could be caused by three different strains of polio; thus, a successful vaccine to prevent polio would need to address all three strains instead of just one. Finally, they documented that the virus reached the nervous tissue, which could cause paralysis, via the bloodstream. This finding suggested that a vaccine could be used to interrupt this path and protect against paralysis. The team used this research to create a vaccine that, when tested in monkeys, protected them from paralysis. The vaccine was tested in 12 children and did raise their polio antibody levels. This was not the vaccine that would later be used in the campaign to eradicate polio; however, both Salk and Sabin did build upon Bodian, Howe, and Morgan's work to develop the two vaccines that are still used to this day.[13]

Another example of the impact that the Johns Hopkins School had includes research on the human papillomavirus, or HPV. For many years, cervical cancer was the leading cause of cancer death in women and was often considered a death sentence. This changed after Dr. Keerti Shah, a professor in molecular microbiology and immunology, discovered through a case-controlled epidemiology study that HPV caused 99.7% of cervical cancers. This finding drove researchers to develop a vaccine, which was approved in 2006.[13] Consequently, cervical cancer morbidity and mortality have been dramatically reduced.

The London School of Hygiene & Tropical Medicine: Established 1922

Satisfied with the creation of an institute of public health in the United States, Rose sought opportunities to create additional institutes of public health. For this, he turned his eyes abroad. Perhaps unsurprisingly, he settled on Britain and the London School of Tropical Medicine.

The History of the London School of Hygiene & Tropical Medicine

The London School of Tropical Medicine, predecessor to the London School of Hygiene & Tropical Medicine, was founded in 1899 by Sir Patrick Manson. He was able to realize his dream of a medical school focused on tropical medicine thanks in part to a donation from philanthropist Bomanjee Dinshaw Petit, as well as financial support from the British Treasury and Colonial Office. Petit, the owner of Petit Mills, a cotton mill, donated £6,666 ($1,368,844 in 2024) to create the school. In a letter to Sir Francis Lovell, then dean of the London School of Tropical Medicine, Petit explained his reasoning:

> This institution, whilst according ample scope to students of diseases that well nigh devastate the East, will be the means of bringing the Western and Eastern minds together to afford help to the suffering East, and thus cementing that union of hearts.[14]

Petit's desire for the London School of Tropical Medicine to address diseases that devastated the East is similar to Rose's idea of public health. However, in saying, "thus cementing the union of hearts," Petit wove into the creation of the school a social and economic context to health that was not seen in Rose's vision of public health. This addition to the London School of Tropical Medicine's mission is evident in its contributions to health, which brought together Rose's biomedical viewpoint and Petit's social and economic context to health.

On October 2, 1899, nineteen years before the Johns Hopkins School of Hygiene and Public Health would open its doors, the London School of Tropical Medicine welcomed 11 students.[15] The school familiarized students with tropical diseases and how to treat them. But it also taught them how to investigate, observe, record, and study diseases. While these skills may not often be the focus of medical students—being more commonly associated with epidemiology—it was only fitting that the London School of Tropical Medicine's students were taught them. The school was located a mere 28 miles from the site where John Snow removed the handle of a water pump during a cholera outbreak in Soho, London, in 1854.[16] By tracing cases and studying who was diagnosed with cholera and who was not, Snow believed that the Broad Street pump was the cause of the cholera outbreak. So, he convinced town officials to let him remove the pump handle, and the cholera outbreak stopped. Snow earned the title of Father of Epidemiology for his work. (However, as the reader will see, in concluding remarks to this chapter, there are others who preceded Snow.)

The London School of Tropical Medicine focused quite heavily on malaria.[15] The school was located at the Albert Dock Seamen's Hospital, which treated former members of the Merchant Navy, fishermen, and their dependents. Given this setting, and the fact that many of these patrons might have been exposed to malaria during their travels, the focus on this disease made sense. Of interest, the school was opposed by the British War Office, the Admiralty, and the medical establishment. The British War Office preferred the Royal Victoria Hospital at Netley as the site for the new school. The medical establishment thought that a new school was unnecessary and that by focusing on tropical diseases, others might think that the many established doctors and physicians practicing in Britain were unable to manage those diseases. It would take some time to convince them that the school itself, as well as its proposed location, were in fact good ideas. Despite opposition, Manson would emerge victorious, establishing the London School of Tropical Medicine at his chosen location. Part of this success was due to the determination of Manson and Herbert Read, the assistant private secretary to Joseph Chamberlain, the colonial secretary of Great Britain at the time. In his post, Chamberlain held a great deal of power. Indeed, his office would provide financial assistance for the founding of the school (£20,000 then, or approximately $4,104,526 in 2024).[17]

In 1913, while Wickliffe Rose was still actively part of the Rockefeller Sanitary Commission for the Eradication of Hookworm Disease and trying to eradicate hookworm in the American South, he consulted Robert Leiper in person at the London School of Tropical Medicine.[18] Leiper was renowned for his work in helminthology (the study of worms), particularly parasitic worms, which include hookworm. Much of his early career was spent traveling through Egypt, Uganda, the Gold Coast, China, and Japan. These trips aided his discoveries, which contributed to knowledge about helminths and their life cycles.[15] While the focus of Rose's visit was not to establish an institute of public health, this visit did serve as the start of the connection between the London School of Tropical Medicine and the Rockefeller Foundation.

The 1918 influenza pandemic brought increased attention to health services in Great Britain, just as it had increased awareness of the need for public health in the United States. As a result, politicians, who were facing increased calls for action, began to understand the need for international vigilance and cooperation and the benefits that this sort of collaboration could provide. To effectively work with other countries, the British Ministry of Health was created in January 1919. This new ministry helped to consolidate the many healthcare activities, which were spread out and separated between different departments, under the control of one ministry.[15]

That same year, Rose attended a meeting of the International Red Cross in Geneva, representing the Rockefeller Foundation's War Relief

Commission.[18] Instead of returning straight to the United Sates, he detoured to Great Britain, where he met with Dr. William Simpson, professor of hygiene and public health in King's College, London.[18] Before returning to Britain, Simpson had served as health officer for Calcutta.[19] Now that the Johns Hopkins School of Hygiene and Public Health had been established and its doors opened, Rose was interested in establishing a sister institute abroad. After his meeting with Simpson on April 20, 1919, Rose wrote that both he and Simpson had a common interest in "establishing a great school of hygiene in London." Rose added that, with the cooperation of the Rockefeller Foundation, Great Britain might "make a monument of victory."[18]

To achieve this, Rose turned to his connection with Leiper, his contact at the London School of Tropical Medicine who he had worked with previously on hookworm eradication. As Leiper was already well connected within the London School, he was able to act as Rose's general adviser in maneuvering the complex world of public health in London. Indeed, it was Leiper who presented Rose with the list of eight centers in Britain that he thought were doing important work in tropical medicine and could work as the home for the school Rose wanted to establish there.[18] The London School of Tropical Medicine was included in Leiper's list.

Much like the process in America, Rose spoke with representatives from the various centers on Leiper's list. The London School, however, was a front-runner. As Rose wrote in a note to himself, the London School of Tropical Medicine and the present Department of Hygiene in University College formed "the nucleus for a future school of hygiene and public health."[18] The use of both "hygiene" and "public health" is interesting, as *hygiene* was used to emphasize a focus on science in regard to health, and *public health*, to emphasize practice and implementation of what students were being taught at the school.

What Rose saw, and others suggested, was that combining the London School of Tropical Medicine and the Department of Hygiene in University College could provide a background in hygiene as well as tropical medicine. Much as Rose highly valued Johns Hopkins's medical school in the decision to establish the first endowed school of public health in the United States, he wanted the school in Great Britain to have access to a medical school as well.

However, Rose ran into some difficulties because many of the individuals he spoke with did not seem to understand his proposal or seemed apathetic about it.[18] While Leiper presented Rose with a proposal to move forward with the development of a program at the London School of Tropical Medicine, nothing came of this idea. Leiper received no response from Rose on the matter. However, seven months after Leiper's letter was sent, he heard from Victor Heiser. Known for his work in leprosy, Heiser was one of Rose's associates at the Rockefeller Foundation.[18]

To Leiper, it probably seemed like no school of public health would be created in Britain with the help of the Rockefeller Foundation because the Rockefeller Foundation had put such discussions on hold. Wanting to focus on the larger picture, the Rockefeller Foundation had decided it did not want to support isolated departments and as such, Leiper's idea to develop a program at the London School of Tropical Medicine was no longer one that it could support. Nonetheless, Leiper continued to help Rose and the Rockefeller Foundation with other work.

This situation changed in 1921, with the recommendations from the Athlone Committee. Named after Alexander Cambridge, the first Earl of Athlone, this committee was created to investigate the needs of physicians and make recommendations to improve health. Among the committee's recommendations were the following:[18]

> An Institute of State Medicine should be established in the University of London in which instruction should be given in Public Health, Forensic Medicine, and Industrial Medicine, and in medical ethics and economics. It should be directly connected with the University of London and under its direct administration ... the income can, in our opinion, be derived from two sources only, state aid and private endowment.

These recommendations cleared the path for the British Ministry of Health to establish the Mond Committee, which was composed of many individuals that Rose had contacted during his original push for a school of public health. Led by Sir Alfred Mond, the minister of health at the time, the Mond Committee concluded that the London School of Tropical Medicine would be the best place to establish this new school of public health. He wrote, "The site should if practicable be contiguous with that of the London School of Tropical Medicine," once again showing the value that he placed on biomedicine.[18]

On February 3, 1922, seven months after the creation of the Mond Committee, Rose and George Edgar Vincent, the president of the Rockefeller Foundation, returned to London. This time, instead of trying to lay the foundations for the idea of a school, they had come to negotiate funding and brought the news that the Rockefeller Foundation wished to provide $2 million for the establishment of said school.[18] This funding would be used to purchase land, such as the Keppel Street site, which still exists to this day, as well as buildings and equipment for the new school. Finally, in February 1924, almost 5½ years after Johns Hopkins School of Hygiene and Public Health opened its doors, the London School of Hygiene & Tropical Medicine was officially formed as a merger of the department of Hygiene in University College and the London School of Tropical Medicine.[15,18]

The Impact of the London School of Hygiene & Tropical Medicine

In 1950, Richard Doll, who was a member of the MRC Statistical Research Unit based at the London School of Hygiene & Tropical Medicine, along with Bradford Hill, who was the director of the Department of Medical Statistics and Epidemiology, published a study that linked smoking with lung cancer. Many studies had associated smoking with lung cancer; however, Doll and Hill's study showed causation between smoking and lung cancer as well as many other diseases.[20] This work was used by advocates to encourage smoking cessation and eventually had a major impact on public health. In the United States, for example, it was a cornerstone of the Food and Drug Administration's "Required Warnings for Cigarette Packages and Advertisements," issued in March 2020.

Maternal mortality, another major public health concern, was addressed in 1989, when Wendy Graham and colleagues from the London School developed the "sisterhood method" to help countries estimate maternal mortality. Using smaller sample sizes than had been used in household surveys, this method made it easier to track the number of women dying due to childbirth, pregnancy, or related causes. The method also allowed for low- and middle-income countries to obtain additional support and funding to address maternal mortality.[21]

Tulane University: The Tulane School of Hygiene and Tropical Medicine: Established 1912

The Tulane School of Hygiene and Tropical Medicine was established without funding from the Rockefeller Foundation four years before the Johns Hopkins school. Thus, it was actually the first established school of public health in the country.

The History

Prior to his role in voting for Johns Hopkins, Abraham Flexner journeyed throughout Europe, visiting schools in Great Britain, France, and Germany. In his book *The American College*, he critiqued the American education system and provided ways to reform education. It was this writing that brought him to the attention of the Carnegie Foundation for the Advancement of Teaching and its head, Henry Pritchett. They were interested in improving medical education as a way to improve healthcare and thus asked Flexner to survey medical schools in the United States and Canada and provide recommendations for improvement.[22]

This report, published in 1910, would become known as the Flexner Report and shape medical education forever.[23] Although Flexner was not a physician, Pritchett and his associates believed that Flexner's findings would be met with less resentment than if they were promoted by a physician. Flexner's report brought about the demise of for-profit proprietary medical schools, as they could not meet the standards he set. It also moved medicine away from alternatives (such as homeopathy and traditional osteopathy) to the evidence-based medical education we see today.[22] As this report was funded and supported by the Carnegie Foundation, it was highly respected and has had lasting ramifications, such as the standardization of medical education.

Unfortunately, Flexner held racist and discriminatory opinions. As a consequence, his report included opinions that led to the closing of the majority of Black medical schools in the United States. This contributed to the paucity of minorities in medicine.[24]

In March 1912, two years after the Flexner Report was published, Dr. Frederick Creighton Wellman, head of the Department of Tropical Medicine and Hygiene at Tulane University, published his paper, "The New Orleans School of Tropical Medicine and Hygiene."[25] This groundbreaking paper highlighted a path to establish a new independent school of public health in the United States; it drew from Wellman's experiences both at the London School of Tropical Medicine and his time in Germany.[26] What was interesting about Wellman's proposal was that the study of hygiene was already established at Tulane University. Indeed, the first formal class on hygiene had been offered by the school, and courses on hygiene had been taught there since 1881.[26]

Wellman had a strong background in both hygiene, which he had taught at the University of California, Berkley, as well as tropical medicine.[26] Before coming to Tulane, he practiced medicine for nine years in Angola, graduated from the London School of Tropical Medicine, and was a professor of tropical medicine at Oakland Medical College in San Francisco.[26] His interest in seeing a school of tropical medicine established in New Orleans was not new, as he had written during his time in San Francisco,

> on account of the diseases brought back from Manila and the Caribbean after the Spanish War, nearly every great port in the United States wanted to become the center of teaching in tropical medicine, New York, New Orleans, and San Francisco being the chief claimants.[27]

While his time in San Francisco did not result in a school of tropical medicine being established there, his time in New Orleans did produce such a result.

The paper he published contained his plans for a school of hygiene and tropical medicine. Included were many statements of support. Flexner wrote, "I believe this effort is distinctly in the interest of science and humanity." Sir Patrick Manson from the London School of Tropical Medicine, the late Surgeon General Walter Wyman, as well as doctors and educators from all over the world, gave support.[25] His plans for instruction were as comprehensive as the various projects he planned for the school to undertake, as well as the various courses the school would offer.

In October 1912, ten months after his paper was published, Tulane established the school of tropical medicine that Wellman so desired. The Tulane board of administrators named him "Professor of Hygiene and Head of the School of Tropical Medicine." Much as how Johns Hopkins and the London School of Hygiene & Tropical Medicine were established due to donations from Petit and Rockefeller, Tulane's School of Hygiene and Tropical Medicine was established thanks to the American Society of Tropical Medicine and a donation of $25,000 (worth about $799,809 in 2024) by Samuel Zemurray.[28] Zemurray would later become president of the United Fruit Company, now known as Chiquita Brands International, and while he had no strong connection to the university, he wished for Tulane to be seen as a great university in his city.[28,29]

In April 1913, Wellman was confirmed as dean of the School of Hygiene and Tropical Medicine by the same board of administrators. Everything Wellman had hoped for was happening. Yet instead of staying at the school and seeing it grow, Wellman eloped with Elsie Dunn to Brazil, leaving his second wife and family behind in the United States.[26] During his time in Brazil, Wellman held a variety of jobs before moving to Europe and becoming a painter and writer under the name of Cyril Kay-Scott.[26] Eventually, he did return to the United States, but he never returned to medicine. Instead, he became the dean of the College of Fine Arts at the University of Denver.[26]

In the midst of Wellman's escapades, the school continued to flourish, even awarding the first Doctor of Public Health degree to Herbert Maxwell Shilstone, as well as the first degree in Tropical Medicine in 1914 to Walton Todd Burres.[26]

Dr. Isadore Dyer and Dr. William H. Seemann attempted to keep the school independent. However, after Wellman's departure, the school was reabsorbed into the School of Medicine, in 1919, and would not become independent again until 1967, under the leadership of Dr. Grace A. Goldsmith.[26] Why is Tulane not seen as the first school of public health in the United States? Because it was reabsorbed into the School of Medicine in 1919, at which point the Johns Hopkins School of Hygiene and Public Health had been accorded that designation.

The Impact of Tulane University

The Tulane School of Hygiene and Tropical Medicine existed for less than a decade. Due to this very short period, many of its alumni have been lost to time and history. Therefore, its importance is that it was technically the first such school.

Concluding Thoughts

BILL FOEGE

The development of schools of public health brought order to the discipline. It resulted in the successful training of people around the world, thus improving the health of all people, not simply those who had access to a medical facility.

Statistics and epidemiology, public health's foundational tools, have been used by some for centuries. But it is only the last 120 years that have made these tools a discipline available to all. There is really no father or mother of epidemiology. John Snow was preceded by Ignaz Semmelweis, in turn preceded by Oliver Wendell Holmes Sr., in turn preceded by Edward Jenner and Alexander Gordon. But that early work was developed into curricula in order to "go to scale."

Flexner, in 1910, changed the future of medical education and is appropriately lauded for that. He made similar contributions to public health education. However, his service is blighted by the racism he espoused. The Flexner Report caused all but two of the seven historically Black medical schools open at the time to be closed. Only Howard University College of Medicine and Meharry Medical College remained open for Black medical students.[30] Over the next 50 years, these two schools would educate 75% of all Black physicians in the United States.[30]

Flexner thought that these two schools were excellent medical schools. However, he believed that Black physicians should only treat patients who were Black and thought that these physicians should not work in the cities but rather return to villages and plantations to serve "their people."[30]

Additionally, Flexner saw Black communities as a "source of infection and contagion." He was concerned that if Blacks lived alongside Whites or treated them, they could infect Whites with hookworm, tuberculosis, or other communicable infectious diseases.[30] He did not see a place for Black doctors in research or academic leadership, but rather he saw them working to maintain the principles of hygiene, sanitation, and civilization. He argued that working in these areas would lead to a decrease in infectious diseases among Black individuals and therefore pose less risk for Whites.[30]

Flexner was supportive of Tulane's development of a school of public health. It is a shame that it faltered—a reminder that maintenance is the foundation of long-term change.

One of the most significant weaknesses of schools of public health is the lack of experience using new tools under the tutelage of instructors. To become a pediatrician, students take care of sick children. To be a surgeon, students practice increasingly difficult surgical techniques. But many public health programs rely on case studies. Schools of public health should take responsibility for providing public health services to designated populations under the guidance of state and local public health programs—and, in so doing, provide students with hands-on public health experience.

This account neglects many recent changes. A large number of US medical schools and schools of public health now have strong programs with other countries. Zoom and other forms of internet-based communication have made daily exchanges of information and problem-solving possible. I recall my surprise, while making rounds in Nairobi, to hear one Kenyan doctor ask another how the University of Washington Huskies had done in the previous day's game!

The National Institutes of Health has provided training and support of medical and public health programs around the world. Countries formerly recipients of assistance are self-reliant in many ways. India, for example, has become a major vaccine producer for the world. In the area of academia, global health has truly become global.

CHAPTER 7

Bilateral Programs

ALISON T. HOOVER

The 2010 earthquake in Haiti killed more than 220,000 people, displaced 1.5 million people, and decimated the health infrastructure. Global health assistance was desperately needed, and nations around the world answered the call. About $13.5 billion in humanitarian aid was pledged, three-quarters of which was from donor nations (the rest was from private charities).[1] Health aid included emergency food assistance, safe drinking water, sanitation systems, shelters, and rebuilding health facilities, as well as scores of volunteer aid workers.[2]

The post-earthquake conditions were dire as water and health infrastructures crumbled. Poor wastewater management at a United Nations peacekeeper camp led to cholera bacteria being introduced into Haiti's largest river, the Artibonite. Hundreds of thousands were infected, and nearly 10,000 died. The outbreak wasn't declared controlled until January 2020, a full decade after the infection was introduced.[3] Controlling the outbreak cost nearly $2.2 billion. As this illustrates, even the most well-intentioned assistance has unanticipated tragedies.

Numerous organizations were involved in the earthquake response. However, a key ingredient was bilateral aid—funding or resources given from one nation to another, such as from the United States directly to Haiti. (By contrast, multilateral aid comes from multiple nations, agencies, or foundations such as the Global Fund for AIDS, Tuberculosis, and Malaria or the World Bank.) Global health funding is often channeled through a mix of bilateral and multilateral programs.

An often-hidden problem with bilateral aid to disaster sites is the cost to the recipient country of being forced to deal with so many agencies at a time when they have other responsibilities. A more perfect approach, almost never reached, would be to have a single person in the country to coordinate all gifts, and a single person outside the country tasked with organizing all donations. The two could coordinate needs, articles received, storage, and distribution.

National health-funding allocations often shift with political winds. Looking at recent US presidents, the George W. Bush and Obama administrations increased the emphasis on multilateral organizations, while the Trump administration favored bilateral approaches. This chapter explores a few of the bilateral programs and their various advantages and weaknesses in promoting global health progress; chapter 8 focuses on multilateral programs.

Bilateral health assistance programs rose to prominence after World War II. One nation supporting another was nothing new, as we saw in chapter 3 on colonial medicine, but such assistance was formalized and organized into dedicated agencies after the war. Bilateral aid does build on colonial roots, in that it is often self-serving and in line with donor nation priorities, thereby perpetuating unequal power dynamics between donor and recipient countries.

The impact of modern bilateral programs is often constrained by dual priorities between domestic policy objectives and health priorities in the countries receiving assistance. For example, it is US law that at least half of transportation companies use US flag–carrying ships to benefit the US economy and fortify the United States's war readiness; this about doubles the overall cost of shipping food aid, adding about $107 million.[4] According to the Government Accounting Office, the cost to send 2,200 tons of US wheat to Ethiopia would cover 5,400 tons of wheat purchased locally. Prioritizing the boost to the donor economy substantially hampers the efficacy of bilateral aid in this instance. Bilateral programs are immensely impactful—2,200 tons of wheat is certainly better than no wheat—but their effectiveness has been hampered by chronic entanglements with national security priorities and political whims.

The program sponsored by the US Agency for International Development (USAID) to eliminate smallpox from 20 countries in West and Central Africa was a success, under budget and faster than expected. But the insistence on American crew cab trucks presented major problems in obtaining parts and knowledgeable mechanics. Using Land Rovers would have benefited the local economy and made the project easier.

Even with its neocolonial approaches, bilateral aid's impact on the global health landscape is momentous. Bilateral programs like USAID's have since allocated billions of dollars in development assistance for health and have had an enormous impact in reducing the spread of HIV, eradicating smallpox, and improving malaria treatment. They have supported the construction of hospitals, the training of healthcare workers, and access to life-saving pharmaceuticals, including those needed to manage HIV. They have had an extraordinary impact on health globally.

US Bilateral Origins

The US approach to foreign aid was shaped dramatically by the two world wars. The United States saw World War I as a war of virtues and labeled its fight for justice, democracy, and peace the model for the world. Foreign assistance in the interwar period focused on technical assistance; providing such knowledge also offered an opportunity to promote American goods and strategic interests. When World War II broke out, foreign aid was quickly coupled with military priorities, as the prominent strategic interest of the time. This coupling continued into the aftermath of World War II—when the priorities for foreign aid were both to contribute to reconstruction and to directly counter Soviet expansion.

The end of World War II saw much of Europe in ruins. Global involvement in the war quickly gave way to global participation in the reconstruction. The United States passed a historic aid package called the Marshall Plan, or the European Recovery Act, in 1948, the same year the World Health Organization (WHO) was founded.

The $15 billion aid package got its name from Secretary of State George C. Marshall, when he included the plan in a speech to Harvard University in June 1947. Marshall didn't write the plan, nor was he first to present it. It was first presented at the Mississippi Teacher's College, written up by young reporter James Reston, and it went nowhere (Bill Foege, pers. comm., 2022). So, the administration pursued a different audience for the plan. The importance of the Harvard speech was not fully acknowledged when it was given; it wasn't even the headline news that day from the university. Actually, the top story of the day was which classes raised the most money for Harvard's endowment.

The Marshall Plan was intended to support Japan and European nations to rebuild infrastructure, bolster economies, overcome trade barriers, and notably, prevent the spread of communism. The soft strategy to counter the rise of communism centered on leveraging foreign aid dollars. The pervasive belief at the time was that communism was best checked through economic growth and strong democratic structures.[5] Billions of dollars were spent on food and raw materials, and policies focused on reducing trade barriers and integrating economies, all with the intent of ameliorating the kind of dire economic conditions in which communism ideals might gain a societal foothold. Some action was a bit more overt—a supplementary US aid package to Italy was conditional on the exclusion of the communist party in the coalition government that Premier Alcide De Gasperi was forming.[6]

The plan wasn't popular, but President Truman and the leaders of the time were confident it was the right thing. This proved to be true, as the reconstruction objectives were accomplished on time and, remarkably, $3.5 billion under budget. The ultimate success of the Marshall Plan opened the door for a sustained, larger-scale effort; the entanglement of foreign policy priorities and international assistance was woven into the foundation of USAID.

USAID was founded in 1961 by President John F. Kennedy through presidential executive order; however, it was not so much something new as it was an aggregation of what had been scattered foreign-assistance efforts up until that point. According to the USAID website, the Mutual Security Agency, Foreign Operations Administration, International Cooperation Administration, Development Loan Fund, and the Food for Peace program, just to name a few, were all subsumed and reorganized under the USAID umbrella at its founding.[7]

President Kennedy founded USAID at a critical moment in global affairs with the explicit intention of advancing America's moral, economic, and strategic interests. But it also marked the introduction of narratives surrounding a moral duty to help. As President Kennedy said:

> The fundamental task of our foreign aid program in the 1960s is not negatively to fight Communism: its fundamental task is to help make a historical demonstration that in the twentieth century, as in the nineteenth—in the southern half of the globe as in the north—economic growth and political democracy can develop hand in hand.[8]

United States Agency for International Development (USAID)

- Founded: 1961
- Money spent on global health in 2019: $12 billion
- Top three thematic areas, in terms of money spent: HIV/AIDS, infectious diseases, and maternal health

One needs to look no further than the stated mission of USAID to see the overtness of the double-barreled priorities of the US bilateral program:

> furthering America's foreign policy interests in expanding democracy and free markets while also extending a helping hand to people struggling to make a better life, recover from a disaster or striving to live in a free and democratic country.[7]

USAID is openly and predominantly guided by US foreign policy interests. Development and humanitarian assistance are central, but secondary, themes; this interwoven mandate has challenged the organization's reputation both domestically and overseas.

USAID's use of global health as a proxy for national defense and diplomacy was cemented by its role in the Vietnam War in the 1960s and 1970s. US involvement in Vietnam was ramping up just as US-AID was established in 1961, resulting in a considerable USAID presence in Vietnam. It was the only country with its own USAID bureau at the time—bureaus are generally organized regionally—and received the largest portion of USAID economic assistance between 1962 and 1975. In 1967, over one-quarter of the entire agency's budget was allocated to Vietnam alone.[9]

This money was funneled into schools, health clinics, hospitals, highways, hydroelectric facilities, industrial centers, and farming cooperatives. Evidence of the blurred line between military strategy and USAID's development assistance was particularly evident in the Chieu Hoi, or "Open Arms," amnesty program it administered that encouraged Viet Cong to desert and join the South Vietnamese cause. The program included job training, political indoctrination, and general integration into South Vietnam, and it was advertised through booklets thrown out of military helicopters or left by soldiers on the battlefield after a firefight.[10,11]

US military strategy in Vietnam went beyond just military prowess to focus on winning "the hearts and minds" of the Vietnamese, the responsibility for which fell to civilian organizations like USAID. The strategy itself was crafted by individuals within the military and the Central Intelligence Agency (CIA), based on a conviction that the war would be won or lost not on the battlefield but in the loyalty of the Southern Vietnamese people. USAID was deemed the vehicle for distributing billions of dollars in aid. Its best-known program was the Civil Operations and Rural Development Support (CORDS) program.

CORDS was one of many "pacification" efforts organized through President Lyndon Johnson's administration to return Viet Cong–controlled areas to South Vietnamese government control. CORDS was the expansion of previous small-scale and generally unsuccessful pacification efforts. Headed by CIA official and National Security

Council member Robert Komer, CORDS was unique in its unification of military, CIA, and USAID efforts under one umbrella program. The CORDS approach was to secure rural areas from Viet Cong–instigated warfare and foster sympathy for the South Vietnamese cause of democracy and its associated freedoms. It ran from 1967 until 1973, when US military and civilian forces were withdrawn.

The program has been criticized for the appropriateness of a pacification program in a war zone. "USAID programs are not built to dig wells and duck bullets at the same time," noted David Reuther, a foreign service officer.[9] But it was also deemed a relative success, in that it did uproot much of the insurgency in South Vietnam that it was originally created to address. Rufus Phillips argues in his memoir, *Why Vietnam Matters: An Eyewitness Account of Lessons Not Learned*, that it was the abandonment of efforts to provide the rural poor with security, opportunities to rise out of poverty, and education on the "merits of democracy and the evils of communism" in 1973 that led to the US defeat in Vietnam.[12]

Komer's own reflection of the CORDS program was that it was "too little, too late."[9] The cause of the US defeat in Vietnam was undoubtedly multifaceted. However, the potential impact of USAID's role in the military conflict set a concerning precedent for the agency as a tool for strategic military interests around the world. Remnants of this role continue to be seen today, such as in Pakistan's polio-eradication efforts.

Fast forward to the late 2000s. USAID partnered with Save the Children to organize a sweeping vaccination campaign for children throughout Pakistan. There was already a decade-long conspiracy theory that polio vaccines were an attempt by the West to sterilize Muslims. As the theory grew in prominence, vaccine hesitancy increased, particularly in militant-stronghold areas in northwest Pakistan, where it borders Afghanistan. It was against this backdrop that Dr. Shakil Afridi began a hepatitis B vaccination campaign in the tribal regions along the Afghan border.[13] He had developed relationships during a USAID and Save the Children seminar. There is still some debate about the original legitimacy of this vaccination campaign, but regardless of its initial intentions, Dr. Afridi was recruited by the CIA to collect DNA from children inside a particularly suspicious compound, while vaccinating from door to door. Although that plan ultimately failed, Dr. Afridi did gather other intelligence during that vaccination visit that led to the midnight May 2, 2011, SEAL team's raid and killing of Osama bin Laden.

When Dr. Afridi's involvement came to light, it added significant fire to the existing hesitancy. The Taliban issued a fatwa (a ruling or statement) against vaccines. What's more, the increased suspicion of healthcare workers administering vaccines has led to the murder of many such workers, disrupted campaigns, and a resurgence of the nearly eradicated virus. The entanglement of US foreign policy and security priorities in the pursuit of bin Laden severely hampered global public health efforts in the region. Some have suggested having USAID's health office report to the Secretary of Health and Human Services instead of the Secretary of State to address the conflation of national security priorities with health activities. The idea has yet to gain traction, likely over political leader reticence to lose health aid as a tool of foreign policy.

At one point during the Nigerian Civil War, during the late 1960s, one of us working in the relief action on the Nigerian side of the line at times relied on military units for support (Bill Foege, pers. comm. 2023). He was never questioned by intelligence officers and learned later that his boss, David Sencer, refused permission when the CIA requested an interview, saying that public health people need to always be trusted to provide healthcare, never military or political variations of that care. It is advice to be recalled by every generation. But, as we will see, the advice must be nuanced.

Though dual priorities of global health and national security have muddled USAID's efficacy, the story of the President's Emergency Plan for HIV/AIDS Relief, or PEPFAR, is indicative of some of the benefits of tethering global health assistance to political priorities. In 2003, President George W. Bush initiated this plan, the largest global health program focused on a single disease in history, because he viewed HIV/AIDS in developing countries as a serious foreign policy concern. The HIV/AIDS epidemic threatened to destabilize the global world order if left unchecked. There was even a UN Security Council session dedicated entirely to HIV in 2000, which marked the first time the Security Council discussed a health issue.[14]

The entanglement of global health objectives with geopolitical politics and foreign policy has mobilized historical amounts of funding. More than $85 billion has been allocated to the global HIV/AIDS response since PEPFAR's establishment. In 2019 alone, according to the *HIV.gov* website, PEPFAR supported HIV testing services for 79.6 million people and antiretroviral treatment for 16.4 million people, contributed to the prevention of 2.6 million cases of mother-to-child HIV transmission, and trained 280,000 health workers. PEPFAR has directly led to sizable increases in the number of people on antiretroviral therapy and to large reductions in mortality.[14] As a huge program with an intensely focused mission, it has transformed the global HIV/AIDS epidemic.

PEPFAR was founded through the United States Leadership Against HIV/AIDS, Tuberculosis, and Malaria Act of 2003, also known as the Global AIDS Act or the Leadership Act. PEPFAR was constructed as a bilateral effort, which represented a departure from the multilateralism that had characterized prior global HIV/AIDS efforts.[15] PEPFAR used a targeted approach in its early years; 15 resource-constrained countries with high HIV/AIDS burdens received $11 billion of the $15 billion in funding. One billion dollars also went to the Global Fund for AIDS, Tuberculosis, and Malaria (hereafter referred to as the Global Fund). PEPFAR funding is implemented through a diverse set of US federal agencies, including USAID, the Office of the Global AIDS Coordinator, Department of Health and Human Services, Centers for Disease Control and Prevention, Department of Defense, Department of Commerce, Department of Labor, and the Peace Corps. It is also common for these agencies to subcontract out, both to other government agencies like the National Institutes of Health and the Food and Drug Administration as well as United States–based nongovernmental organizations such as FHI 360, PATH, and Population Services International. PEPFAR is accountable to the US Congress and reports on an annual basis.

PEPFAR's bilateral approach has occasionally been criticized as replacing support for multilateral commitments, such as to the Global Fund. A counterargument has been that multilateral programs do not wield the same leverage in urging large-scale national-level health reforms, making bilateral programs a more effective mechanism for long-term change. Although a greater share of PEPFAR funding has been allocated to multilateral programs recently, PEPFAR does have a cap on its multilateral allocations, known as the one-third cap. PEPFAR regulations limit US contributions to the Global Fund: they are not to exceed 33% of all funds donated to the Global Fund by all donors during a specified period. Any contributions withheld due to this regulation are to be redirected to bilateral programs.

In another example of tethering political objectives to health priorities, Global Fund commitments have a further limitation. If the Global Fund allocates resources to country governments known to support repeated "acts of international terrorism," an equivalent monetary amount is withheld from US contributions the following fiscal year.[16] According to an Office of Inspector General report, for fiscal years 2009–2011, this was applied to Cuba, Iran, Sudan, and Syria.

Withholding health aid as a form of political leverage can be problematic. Though it is logical to want to avoid supporting countries that sponsor terrorism, hinging health financing on such terms ultimately hurts those living in the country more than those who run it. The challenge for bilateral programs is to design programs that maintain vitally needed health support that can continue in the face of political friction and ideology misalignment. Politically guided approaches are rarely aligned with health-guided approaches.

In addition to political priorities, PEPFAR's programming has also been vulnerable to impositions of morality at the expense of approaches with proven impact. PEPFAR offers no funding for needle-exchange programs, despite their proven effectiveness as a critical HIV-prevention tool. One-third of prevention spending in 2006–2008 went toward abstinence-only programs, although one study suggested the $1.3 billion spent on abstinence-only education in sub-Saharan Africa had no impact.[17] Though it is no longer a requirement to allocate a specific amount to abstinence-only programming, there is continued emphasis on including such messaging. A report must be submitted to Congress if less than half of prevention funds are spent on abstinence, delay of sexual initiation, monogamy, fidelity, and partner-reduction activities in any host country with a generalized epidemic.[16] The original 2003 PEPFAR legislation also mandated an anti-prostitution pledge, where no funds could be made available to "any group that does not have a policy explicitly opposing prostitution and sex trafficking." This hampered outreach with sex workers. That pledge was thrown out in the Supreme Court in 2013 as a First Amendment violation, but a provision still lingers stipulating that no funds may be used to promote or advocate for the legalization or practice of prostitution.[18]

PEPFAR is a powerful example of the benefits and shortcomings of entangling political priorities with global health assistance. The need to address foreign policy concerns around the rapidly growing HIV/AIDS epidemic in the early 2000s led to billions of dollars of support for testing and treatment. Plus, this HIV assistance coalesced partnerships, funding, and commitments around global public health in general, creating enormous momentum for global health assistance on the whole. Governments and their bilateral programs can thus mobilize almost unparalleled amounts of funding for global health.

Nonetheless, as with the Ethiopian food aid example, money is rarely spent in a way that maximizes efficiency and impact on health outcomes, because of the need to balance economic and foreign policy priorities. With PEPFAR, much of the funding goes to stand-alone programs for HIV testing and counseling as opposed to strengthening overall health systems. The program has generated colossal support and money for HIV/AIDS programming, but without commensurate improvements across other global health indicators, such as in maternal and child health or diarrheal diseases. PEPFAR's concentrated focus on HIV/AIDS is potentially at the direct expense of other health issues. PEPFAR pays local health workers up to 100 times what they make in the domestic health system. This system ultimately taps into a finite pool of skilled medical professionals and disincentivizes them to work within the domestic healthcare system.[19]

PEPFAR illuminates the power of governments and their bilateral programs to rally global commitment and mobilize enormous financial resources. It also highlights opportunities to steer programs to be more effective in improving overall population health.

Global Affairs Canada

- Founded: 1968 (known then as Canadian International Development Agency)
- Money spent on global health in 2019: $1.1 billion
- Top three thematic areas, in terms of money spent: child health, maternal health, and strengthening of sector-wide approaches and health systems

Canada's overseas health assistance reflects long-standing national strategies of multilateralism and global citizenship. As a global "middle power," Canada has relied on partnerships and consensus building since its establishment as a nation, when it called on the United Kingdom and France to fend off US attempts to annex British Columbia during the gold rush of the 1850s and 1860s. The United States was very intent on expanding its territory, having just acquired land from Mexico in 1848 and purchased Alaska in 1867. The discovery of gold in British Columbia fanned these flames, until the area was confederated into Canada in 1871.

Canada's continued emphasis on partnerships is evident in its health aid mechanisms. Health assistance allocations to multilateral agencies such as WHO and the Global Fund have increased in the last decade. Canada does have a bilateral program, which has undergone a series of reorganizations and is now known as Global Affairs Canada, since 2013. Global Affairs Canada and its predecessor, the Canadian International Development Agency, were the most prominent health assistance funding mechanism for the Canadian government from 1997 to 2008. Canadian bilateral assistance has traditionally focused on strengthening national health systems, gender equity, environmental health, maternal health, and reproductive health.

While Global Affairs Canada continues to represent a major portion of Canada's funding, its total share has declined since 2010. Its contribution is now spread more evenly across multilateral agencies and nongovernmental organizations (NGOs). In part, this reflects Canada's expanded support for multilateral initiatives such as the G8 Muskoka Initiative for Maternal, Newborn, and Child Health. This initiative disburses funding through multilateral organizations, UN agencies, and international NGOs. It is also a reflection of a foreign policy stance of prioritizing Canada's competitive position during Prime Minister Stephen Harper's administration. Harper, who took power in 2006, reduced overall development assistance but actually increased funding for health assistance as part of projecting Canada as a major global power. The Harper administration's efforts to link Canada's economic policy and trade priorities with foreign development are most visible through the creation of Global Affairs Canada; it merged the Canadian International Development Agency and the Department of Foreign Affairs and International Trade to align aid with trade and investment interests.[20]

The election of Justin Trudeau and his liberal party in 2015 set a more progressive tone for Canada's overseas health assistance. In June 2017, Trudeau announced the Feminist International Assistance Policy, making it only the second country after Sweden to have an explicitly named feminist foreign policy.[21] The policy uses a rights-centered approach to international assistance, which focuses on six priority areas: gender equality and the empowerment of women and girls, human dignity, growth that works for everyone, environment and climate action, inclusive governance, and peace and security.[22] The policy came with an additional $3.5 billion investment on top of previous international assistance commitments.[23] A unique feature of the investments included a $650 million allocation for sexual and reproductive health and rights, which then grew to a $1.4 billion commitment.[24]

The focus on sexual and reproductive health marked a significant change in administrative priorities from the Harper administration. That administration limited sexual and reproductive health programs to family planning. The Trudeau administration funding is geared toward comprehensive sexuality education, sexual and gender-based violence, female genital mutilation, and the right to choose safe and legal abortion alongside access to post-abortion care.[24] Global Affairs Canada's earmarked funding for sexual and reproductive health, particularly abortion access and care, was critically needed in the global health landscape. Canada played an essential balancing role in filling the vacuum created when the Trump administration reimposed the Mexico City policy that barred any groups that provided abortion counseling, services, or care from being eligible for US funding.

Broadly, Canada has emerged as a leader in promoting gender equity as a central tenet of overseas assistance, particularly under the Trudeau government. The Feminist International Assistance Policy aims to have at least 95% of Canada's bilateral international assistance spending target gender equity and the empowerment of women and girls by 2021–2022.[22] The policy has been well-received by NGOs, governments, and UN agencies.[25]

Global Affairs Canada and its predecessors have faced their own set of critiques. Canada is a major financial player in the bilateral health program world, but its global contributions are low relative to its gross national income. As Canada has developed and advanced, it has not allocated proportional funding to global development on the whole, though its commitments, to health in particular, have been increasing in recent years. The consolidation of the Canadian International Development Agency and the Department of Foreign Affairs and International Trade to become Global Affairs Canada in 2013 also raised concerns in the global community about tying international health assistance to Canadian trade and investment interests.

As a result, Canada's bilateral program has been subject to complaints similar to those leveled at its American counterpart. Defense and diplomacy guide decision-making rather than health priorities, leading to limited health impact. Canada's languid Disaster Assistance Response Team (DART) effort after the 2005 earthquake in Kashmir, Pakistan, was a vivid example of the challenges in conflating national defense and global health.

DART was a military project designed to rapidly deploy anywhere in the world for any number of crises and emergencies. Yet DART's Kashmir response took 14 days to be fully operational, and ultimately their 6 physicians, 2 physician assistants, 5 registered nurses, 30 medical technicians, and 60 armed soldiers treated 11,782 people and cost over $15 million. They were slow to operationalize, costly, and had limited impact. The DART response was criticized for lending too much attention to technological solutions, at the expense of local primary care needs. This criticism was not new, having been expressed during the 1985 response to the Mexico City earthquake and the 2004 tsunami in the Asia-Pacific region.[26]

In summary, Global Affairs Canada and its predecessor have been linchpins in alliance building and global multilateral health initiatives. Recently, it also been a global leader in promoting gender equity and sexual health initiatives. Yet, like its US counterpart, the Canadian bilateral program's entanglement of health assistance with defense, trade, and investment interests has constrained its effectiveness.

Cuba Medical Internationalism

- Began: 1959
- Money spent on global health in 2016: $12.8 million[27]

To draw a contrast to Canada's delays, Cuba's bilateral program was significantly more effective in the Kashmir response. Cuba had 173 physicians and support staff on the ground within 72 hours. By the time DART was operational, Cuba already had 600 health professionals on the ground. Cuba's team members had completed the construction of several field hospitals and were traveling to provide care in remote areas. By the end of their 13-month involvement, 1,481 physicians and 900 paramedics served in Pakistan, treating over 1 million patients.

Cuba provides more medical personnel to the developing world than all of the G8 nations (France, Germany, Italy, the United Kingdom, Japan, the United States, Russia, and Canada) combined. And, as a notable indication of Cuba's emphasis on sustainability, the Cuban Ministry of Health also offered 1,000 medical scholarships for young Pakistanis to receive free medical training in Cuba to carry on the work the Cuban health professionals had begun.

Cuba's internationalism has its roots in anti-imperialist Marxist-Leninist ideologies during Fidel Castro's tenure in the 1960s, which seeped into the country's global health approach.[28] Cuba's first international health aid was a medical brigade of 55 doctors and nurses to Algeria in 1963 during its war for independence from the French. Cuba has since provided medical assistance to more than 100 countries worldwide, many of which it is ideologically at odds with. Cuba has managed to build cooperative foreign relations by using its overseas development assistance money to focus on global health, addressing immediate humanitarian needs, and building recipient country capacity to meet health challenges. It appears that Cuba, while not ignoring its own foreign policy ambitions, is instead advancing them in a more subtle and perhaps more effective way than the US and Canadian bilateral programs.

Although Cuba has not prioritized its political agenda over its health aid, it may have prioritized its economy. One of the sharpest critiques of Cuba's health aid is its industrialization; Cuba's overseas medical teams are a major source of income for the island nation. Many of its international agreements involve a direct payment to the Cuban government for sending its doctors, with only a small share allocated directly to the doctors themselves. Under the Mais Médicos program in Brazil, the Cuban government pocketed three-quarters of Brazil's monthly payments to the doctors.[29] Human rights concerns have been raised about the low salaries Cuba affords its overseas medical providers, alongside coercion and surveillance. USAID even put out a call for applications in 2019 for organizations to track and measure human rights violations among overseas Cuban medical professionals, which was quickly and thoroughly denounced by the Cuban government.[30] Even the host countries have qualms about Cuban medical teams; some medical associations in health team–recipient nations have also complained about the utility and appropriateness of bringing in foreign health professionals when many local health workers remain unemployed.

Underscoring the human rights concerns, scores of Cuban healthcare providers have defected from Cuba while serving on overseas medical teams. Many came to the United States from 2006 to 2017 through the Cuban Medical Professional Parole program, which fast-tracked visas for medical professionals and their families. Some criticized the program as immoral for encouraging a medical "brain drain" from under-resourced countries; others called it necessary humanitarianism.[31]

Cuba's approach appears to be lengthy in-country stays, heavy investment in local capacity-building and fostering of long-term stability, and a focus on long-standing cooperation as opposed to short-term endeavors. The country's health aid approach has been generally effective and impactful, but it is laden with costs for its own health workers and appears to be unduly influenced by economic priorities.

Swedish International Development Agency (Sida)

- Founded: 1965
- Money spent on global health in 2019: $720 million
- Top three thematic areas, in terms of money spent: maternal health, child health, and HIV/AIDS

Sweden is another success story on the bilateral stage. Though not a mighty donor in terms of crude capital, Sweden has set itself apart as the top donor, when measured as a percentage of GDP (gross domestic product; compared to Canada, for example). Sweden is also remarkable for its strong governmental commitment to global health assistance. This social and political commitment is predicated on a concept called *Sverigebilden*, or the view of Sweden in the world that is promoted by the Swedish government. Sweden views itself as a provider of welfare both at home and abroad, leading to generous development aid commitments and posing challenges for any political party seeking to reduce aid budgets.[32]

Even with this political security, or perhaps because of it, Sida has also made concerted efforts to divorce itself from politics, including going so far as to go against the wishes of its umbrella ministry, the Ministry for Foreign Affairs. Toward the end of the Smallpox Eradication Initiative in the 1970s, the Ministry for Foreign Affairs grew concerned that the focus on smallpox was too disease specific and not tied to broader health system strengthening. In spite of this, Sida leadership was convinced of the initiative's importance. Not only did Sida continue funding it, but it was the only group to provide unconditional funding, which proved critical in the eradication effort.

Sweden also has two elements that bolster the credibility of its bilateral program. First, the country emphasizes solidarity in its programming and strives to implement similar things at home and abroad. Second, Sweden's neutrality during the world wars and its general non-aligned, non-colonial status greatly diminishes suspicion on the part of host countries regarding subtle political interference.

Ultimately, it is Sweden's credibility, apolitical assistance history, and historical neutrality that lends itself to generally successful bilateral assistance.

China International Development Cooperation Agency (CIDCA)

- Founded: 2018
- Money spent on global health in 2019: $730 million
- Top three thematic areas, in terms of money spent: sector-wide approaches and health systems strengthening, infectious diseases, and child health

Although China's bilateral agency is nascent—it was founded in 2018—its overseas health assistance is not. China dispatched its first medical team to Algeria in 1963, around the same time Sweden, Canada, and US bilateral programs were launching, and identical to Cuba's early international medical team assistance. China is unique in that it was both a recipient of global health donor funds and a donor of global health aid for many decades. Its income per capita and disease burden rates did not formally exceed levels for graduation from Global Fund support until 2014, though China's receipt of health funds became controversial in the late 2000s. Debate over its recipient status flourished after China spent $46 billion on hosting the 2008 Olympic Games, compounded by a $586 billion economic stimulus package the same year.[33] Funding was also suspended in 2011 after China failed to meet monitoring requirements and an audit revealed the nation was not giving the stipulated 35% of an AIDS grant to community-based organizations. Funding was resumed later that year.

When it comes to development assistance, healthcare isn't China's focus; infrastructure is.[34] But the health assistance China does offer focuses more on health system strengthening than on disease-specific programs—sometimes called vertical programs. The most typical form of China's health assistance is dispatching Chinese medical teams, likely a reflection of their highly effective domestic community health worker system. Originally called "barefoot doctors" in 1968–1985, and "village doctors" since then, the system encompasses a large cadre of individuals equipped with basic medical training to address health disparities in rural areas. Approximately 1.5 million community health workers have received brief but intensive traditional and modern medical training since 1968 and have become the mainstay of rural health in China.[35] In the early days of the program, participating barefoot doctors also served as key revolutionary emblems for China's Cultural Revolution. The community health worker devotion to improving rural access to healthcare was commonly evoked in propaganda as part of the militarization of civilians and has resulted in a complicated legacy for the program.[36] Nevertheless, China's community health worker system was effective in bringing basic health services to rural and underserved areas, which is a critical and persistent need in modern global health assistance.

According to national statistics, from 2010 to 2012, China sent 3,600 medical staff to 54 countries and treated approximately 7 million patients. China has taken a similar approach with global COVID-19 response, sending medical teams and personal protective equipment (PPE) supplies across Asia, Europe, Africa, and North and South America.[37]

Aligned with its major influence on health system strengthening, other health assistance has included building health facilities, donating medical equipment and drugs, and training local healthcare workers.

There is one disease China's health assistance has focused on: malaria. This may be in part due to the country's success in controlling malaria domestically and its substantial contributions to antimalarial pharmaceuticals.

The compound artemisinin—the foundation for antimalarials and treatment regimens around the world—was discovered by Chinese researcher Tu Youyou in 1972. It is an extract from the Artemisia annual plant, which had been used in traditional Chinese medicine for centuries to treat fevers.[38,39] Along with artemisinin, China's overseas health assistance continues to use traditional medicinal approaches, including acupuncture, naprapathy, and herbal medicines, despite the lack of randomized control trials evidencing impact.

Assistance from China often faces suspicions of its true intentions. China is one of the top-10 bilateral donors to the African continent. Official national statistics suggest that more than half of China's global aid is allocated to the African continent (again, healthcare is not the most important component of China's foreign aid). China's interest in collaboration with the African continent was likely grounded in economic opportunity; the continent's raw natural resources hold great, and profitable, opportunities for manufacturing-centric China.

China's economic expansion relies on its production of manufactured goods, necessitating raw materials. The African continent is rich in raw materials but needs stronger infrastructure to effectively develop and capitalize on its natural resources. China's own development story hinged upon successful infrastructure, making it an appealing partner for African nations. Their complementary needs and opportunities have led to an exponential growth in economic investments from China in recent years. China's foreign direct investment increased 9000% from $491 million in 2003 to an astounding $44.3 billion in 2019, surpassing the United States in 2014.[40]

As recent evidence of the ongoing convergence of economic interests and health diplomacy on the African continent, the cost of China's

COVID-19 aid to Algeria and Nigeria was underwritten by Chinese state-owned enterprises operating in the respective nations, rather than the central government. In Algeria, the China State Construction Engineering Corporation footed the bill for a 13-member medical relief team, supplies including PPE and respirators, and the construction of a local hospital.[41]

Yet investment trends seem to reflect both development and national interest, and funding is not constrained to just resource-rich nations. China may have come for the economic opportunity, but it has reaped major benefits in support for its foreign policy objectives of countering Western influence and bolstering the One China policy at the expense of Taiwan and Tibet. China has branded its global health assistance as an altruistic counterbalance to US power and an alternative to the Western model of development.

Unlike the Washington Consensus—a set of economic policies that form the structure of reform packages promoted by the International Monetary Fund, World Bank, and US Government agencies—China's aid has no requirements of good governance, democracy, or respect for human rights. In China's view, this offers more of a "no strings attached" approach to overseas aid as it is deemed unconditional on accounts of morality or democracy, but rather is guided by a responsibility to support developing countries. According to China's Eight Principles for Economic Aid and Technical Assistance, which guide its overseas aid portfolio, China's foreign aid approach with partner countries, such as within Africa, is guided by principles of noninterference with domestic affairs of a recipient country, mutual benefits, and self-determination.[42]

While China may not interfere with the domestic affairs of a recipient country, it is in some ways asking recipient countries to interfere with China's domestic affairs around the One China policy. This was especially true in the 1980s and 1990s, when China suspended medical cooperation and withdrew its medical personnel from nations that had diplomatic relations with Taiwan, and only resumed cooperation upon the termination of such relations. This one string in its otherwise no-strings-attached approach is a sizeable string, as support for the One China policy from African nations bolstered China's stance against Taiwan's application for a seat at the United Nations. Taiwan still does not have its own seat. No matter how altruistic the original intentions may have been, China's overseas health aid is certainly functioning as a soft power mechanism for economic opportunity and political agendas, including countering Western dominance.

In addition to critiques of its opportunism in the African continent, CIDCA faces significant criticism for its lack of transparency in data and accountability. Before CIDCA was founded, China's health aid was managed by the ministry of commerce, with support from other ministries, departments, and bureaus. National-level agencies initiated and negotiated agreements, but implementation usually fell to provincial or subnational governments. This decentralization, coupled with interprovincial competition, limited the coordination and cohesion of China's health aid; the amount of resources allocated to projects tended to reflect specific provincial capacity, rather than the need of recipient projects and areas.

The lack of national oversight and coordination has hindered reporting. Little is known about the scope, effectiveness, or governance of China's health aid, nor how priorities and allocations of health aid are determined. There are no mechanisms from either China or recipient nations to determine the amount or impact of aid. Most countries transitioning from recipient to donor countries do not report to international aid depositories, and China is no exception. As a result, China's role as a global health donor is generally unquantified, especially in comparison to other major donors. China has made various commitments to address these gaps in data, but it has yet to result in concrete findings.

This lack of transparency may be intentional. Should China reveal the extent of its foreign aid, it could open itself to criticism about overseas commitments while chronic poverty persists within its own borders. It may also desire to avoid the appearance of favoritism with specific countries, since it has branded itself as a more altruistic dispenser of aid than other bilateral programs. Yet there is a cost to this obscurity, principally through mistrust and suspicion on the part of recipients. The lack of monitoring and accountability also constrains the overall impact of its health aid portfolio.

Recipient populations of China's aid in Africa seem to exhibit a blend of appreciation, support, suspicion, and ultimately resignation to the growing power of China in their local economy and geopolitical priorities. Nigerian Health Minister Osagie Ehanire's announcement in early April 2020 that he had invited an 18-person medical team from China to assist in the local COVID-19 response yielded swift backlash from professional and medical organizations. They decried the need for foreign experts, citing the skills and abilities of Nigerian healthcare workers (again with the Cuban parallels).[41] The Nigerian Union of Journalists also went so far as to suggest that the Chinese medical team could be using Nigerians as "guinea pigs" for experiments while also expressing anti-Chinese sentiments and conspiracy theories that bringing in Chinese workers could lead to a spike in the virus's prevalence in the country.[43]

Few of these sentiments were new; one interviewee in a study of attitudes among those working directly with Chinese health aid programs in Malawi and Tanzania said, "You [China] just came here to build, just making money here, has not brought benefits to the locals. This is why they took Africa as a new colony." While most participants had a deep appreciation for the aid and the overall China–Africa cooperation, they identified frustrations and opportunities to improve in culturally specific communication, power imbalances, aid program organization and management, and sustainability.[44]

China seems to represent a new approach to bilateral programs, with its own successes and shortcomings. With the relatively recent establishment of a coordinated bilateral entity, new management and coordination priorities could reshape China's health aid in coming years. It remains to be seen what kind of outcomes its assistance is producing, but there's no question China is one to watch going forward.

Key Lessons

Bilateral programs are as complex as the geopolitical environments in which they exist. Drawing from the lessons of the United States, Canada, Cuba, Sweden, and China, the most effective bilateral health programs maintain a form of independence from political leaders. The independence can entail being an independent agency; instituting a policy and financial buffer from swings in political administration changes and the resulting priority re-directions; or simply instituting concrete, long-term funding allocations. Effective interventions and activities from bilateral programs have focused on long-term health system strengthening, building local capacity through technical assistance, and playing to a nation's comparative strengths. Going forward and in the wake of COVID-19's global echo, the best global health assistance may not center on bilateral programs, so much as on collaborative multilateral programs.

Concluding Thoughts

BILL FOEGE

Bilateral programs have had astounding results in providing resources, garnering political support, and increasing local participation. At their best, they provide effective and efficient programs that also improve the relationships between countries. At its worst, bilateralism uses health assistance to promote political agendas; encourages inefficiency, when equipment and supplies must come from the donor country; and raises all of the unequal status concerns that infected colonialism.

As a reviewer has pointed out, just as church-sponsored programs often succumbed to the use of medical programs as an enticement to join the sponsoring church groups, so also are health assistance programs so attractive that it was inevitable that countries would use such bilateral aid to encourage coalitions with other countries.

It is very difficult to resist such forces and provide approaches that are positive, fair, and driven by a focus on the health of recipients.

CHAPTER 8

Multilateral Organizations

ALISON T. HOOVER AND MADISON GABRIELLA LEE

Unlike bilateral organizations, many programs involve multiple sponsoring countries, corporations, academic institutions, foundations, and the like. While their management is often difficult, they provide advantages because many are invested in a common endeavor and funding may be easier to obtain. It is impossible, in this chapter, to cover the plethora of such programs, so we will focus on some of the oldest, best-known, or intriguing multilateral organizations.

World Health Organization (WHO)

WHO Director-General Dr. Tedros Adhanom Ghebreyesus sought to declare the novel coronavirus a public health emergency of international concern on January 23, 2020. Reluctant to act prematurely after criticism that WHO overreacted to the H5N1 pandemic, the declaration was delayed for another week—after nearly 8,000 confirmed cases of COVID-19 and more than 200 deaths had occurred. The day the declaration was announced, Tedros praised China for its transparency and quick action to control the spread of the infection, saying the Chinese were "setting a new standard for outbreak response."[1]

Criticisms of China and WHO mounted over the subsequent months, when it became clear that Chinese authorities delayed reporting the novel coronavirus to WHO. Chinese authorities also suppressed information on human-to-human transmission, insisting transmission was limited to animal exposure—until reports from other nations provided evidence to the contrary. Questions persist about the accuracy of the early data China released, and Tedros's early praise for China's transparency quickly became a flash point for the WHO's leadership in the pandemic.[2]

The US Government was a particularly vocal critic of WHO early in the outbreak, calling the agency too slow to sound the alarm and too deferential to the Chinese government. President Donald Trump announced a pause on US funding for WHO in April 2020 to investigate its "mismanagement of the coronavirus pandemic," and ultimately submitted notice of the US decision to withdraw from membership in WHO in July 2020.[3] On his first day in office, President Joe Biden reversed the decision, citing the multilateral agency as playing "a crucial role in the world's fight against the deadly COVID-19 pandemic as well as countless other threats to global health and health security."[4]

WHO is vulnerable to such rapid transitions between currying global favor and serving as a scapegoat, due in part to its broad and nonspecific mandate. That mandate, when WHO was formed in 1948 as the first United Nations specialized multilateral agency, was to "act as the directing and co-ordinating [sic] authority on international health work."[5] Initially, WHO assumed the responsibilities of the League of Nations and the United Nations Relief and Rehabilitation Administration, including classifying diseases and causes of death as well as the epidemiologic notification service.[6] Priority health issues for the agency in 1948 focused on communicable diseases such as malaria, sexually transmitted diseases, and tuberculosis, alongside maternal and child health, nutrition, and environmental health. WHO has also been a central source of accurate data on the prevalence of global morbidity and mortality. The organization continues to serve similar but evolved functions today. It sets international standards for case definitions and treatment, offers a global standard for drug approvals, provides guidance on important health issues, and coordinates responses to health emergencies like COVID-19.

Before COVID-19, WHO contributed to a number of major global health achievements. In 1978, WHO and UNICEF cosponsored the International Conference on Primary Health Care to promote understanding and adoption of primary healthcare, which was at the time a nascent and novel concept.[7] Up to that point, medicine and healthcare principally consisted of doctors and hospitals. The barefoot doctor movement in China (see chapter 7) was hugely formative in the primary healthcare movement, with its emphasis on prevention rather than cure and the provision of basic services at the community level.[8] WHO and UNICEF sought to reach consensus on a global declaration by building upon several national, regional, and international meetings that had been held on primary healthcare.

Delegations from 134 countries and 67 United Nations organizations attended the conference, held in Almaty (formerly Alma-Ata) in present-day Kazakhstan September 6–12, 1978. The resulting declaration from the conference, known as the Declaration of Alma-Ata, affirmed the right to health for all, acknowledged the role of social determinants in health, decried health inequality, and emphasized the role of primary healthcare in addressing health inequality.[7] The Alma-Ata declaration, radical and groundbreaking for its time, was endorsed by all WHO member states. WHO served an important function in creating global consensus and ushering in a new era of healthcare. Its coordination and global health leadership, in tandem with UNICEF, generated broad commitments from the governments of member nations to promulgate primary healthcare as national policy. Of course, implementing such a broad declaration has posed its own challenges, but the consensus that emerged from Alma-Ata created a critical impetus to explore health holistically and focus on equity and social determinants.[9]

WHO also sponsored and promoted the ultimate eradication of smallpox. Smallpox was one of the most devastating diseases known to humanity, with around 50 million cases each year, before vaccinations were available, and a mortality rate of about 30%.[10] Smallpox killed Queen Mary II of England, King Luis I of Spain, Tsar Peter II of Russia, and King Louis XV of France, to name just a few of its high-profile victims. In the 18th century, every seventh child in Russia died of smallpox.

Armed with a highly effective vaccine, WHO launched a global eradication campaign in 1967. As a result of a well-coordinated effort by WHO, the last case of endemic smallpox was reported in 1977. Global eradication was certified and endorsed by the World Health Assembly (the decision-making body of WHO) in 1980. The effort to eradicate smallpox is largely considered one of the most successful and most collaborative public health initiatives in history.

In 2003, WHO negotiated its first international treaty: the WHO Framework Convention on Tobacco Control. The treaty was developed in response to the global tobacco epidemic and represented a paradigm shift in using regulation to address addictive substances. The framework convention also addressed some of the critical questions of liability and accountability. It ultimately became one of the most rapidly and widely embraced treaties in United Nations history.[11] Studies have shown that the framework convention was markedly successful in contributing to the development and implementation of tobacco-control policy, and that countries that implemented the framework convention at higher levels had greater reductions in smoking prevalence.[12,13] This convention gave countries legal footing to stand on against the tobacco industry and helped identify interference by the tobacco industry.[14]

More recently, WHO's 2019–2023 general program of work focused on expanding universal health coverage, addressing health emergencies (prescient), and promoting well-being, not merely the absence of disease, as a goal.[15] This program was designed to facilitate health components of the Sustainable Development Goals and to prioritize reducing health inequities.

Over the last seven decades, the growth in WHO's scope has gravely outpaced increases in its budget. The organization is funded through member states' dues and voluntary contributions. Its 2022–2023 operating budget was $6.7 billion over the two years. By contrast, the US CDC budget request for just fiscal year 2023 is $10.675 billion.[16,17] Less than $1 billion of WHO's budget comes from set member states' dues, underscoring WHO's reliance on voluntary contributions to make up nearly 90% of its budget.[16] The United States is historically the single largest contributor to WHO, though funding withheld during the Trump administration in 2020–2021 caused the United States to cede its customary top-donor position to Germany.[18] As the (usual) largest contributor, the United States's funding pause had the potential to be very impactful had it not been reversed, raising questions about the leverage that the United States has to influence WHO policy. Many of the voluntary contributions are also earmarked for specific activities by the donors, constraining WHO's flexibility and coordinating power.[19] For context, about two-thirds of the US contributions are voluntary.

Without flexible funding sources, WHO faces greater challenges to respond to emerging health concerns, such as Ebola or COVID-19. Facing criticism after an Ebola outbreak in 2014–2015, the agency did establish a Health Emergencies Programme and a Contingency Fund for Emergencies.[20] But neither of these mechanisms was designed to address a lasting global pandemic like COVID-19.

Another key constraint to WHO's effectiveness has been its need to respond to divisive geopolitical tensions in the ways they influence health. The World Health Assembly made explicit statements affirming Palestine's right to a sovereign state and acknowledging that the Israeli occupation poses serious health problems.[21] By the same hand, WHO has also been accused of ignoring the impacts of other geopolitical conflicts, such as in Syria.[22]

As evidence of the way political interference damages WHO's effectiveness, WHO cannot share information with Taiwan because that country is not a member of the United Nations. (The same applies to the International Olympics Committee and the International Civil Aviation Organization.)[23] As discussed in greater detail in the bilateral programs chapter, this is in part due to support from African aid-recipient nations for the One China policy. Taiwan sits just 100 miles off the east coast of China and had some of the first coronavirus cases outside of China, but it did not have access to vital epidemiologic information from WHO during the pandemic.

Taiwan's exclusion from WHO was also detrimental during the SARS epidemic in 2003, when Taiwan was not able to participate in WHO's global outbreak alert and response system. Taiwan attempted to report suspected cases to WHO, but the cases were not included in WHO data for several days. When the data were eventually added, the cases were only attributed to Taiwan as a province of China.[24] WHO also did not provide Taiwan scientists with virus samples to support vaccine and treatment research, nor did it deploy experts to assist in containment efforts.[25]

Although it can withhold information, WHO ultimately holds no enforcement authority with its health guidance. It cannot bind, censure, or sanction its member nations. The organization is designed to earn its legitimacy through its scientific expertise.[26] But when WHO guidance was not adhered to during the ongoing COVID-19 pandemic, the organization had no methods of recourse.

The global nature of the pandemic has laid plain the need for coordinated responses to global health threats—as well as the cost of uncoordinated and underfunded response agencies.

World Bank

It may come as a surprise that the current largest funder of health within the United Nations system is not WHO, but the World Bank.[27] Though not traditionally considered a player in global health, the World Bank was one of the first and largest donors in the global COVID-19 response. A month after the outbreak was first declared a pandemic, the World Bank had allocated $6 billion to WHO and to direct strengthening of national health systems, which amounted to nearly one-third of all funds mobilized at that point.[28] Nor was COVID-19 the World Bank's first foray into global health programs. It surpassed WHO in terms of funding in the late 1990s and has continued to make significant increases to its health portfolio in the last two decades.[27,29]

As with many of the major bilateral programs, the World Bank was founded in 1944 to support effective post–World War II reconstruction. Its first grant was to France in 1947 for equipment and raw materials.[30] Over time, the link between a healthy population and a healthy economy became impossible to ignore. In 1985, less than 1% of World Bank spending was on health, but today it is closer to 12% annually.[27]

The World Bank's expanded investments in health financing can be traced back to when Dr. Jim Yong Kim became president of the World Bank in 2012. Kim was the first physician to be president of the World Bank, in itself a statement on the importance of health in economic growth and productivity. It came as a surprise to many when Kim was nominated, both because he had not been publicly mentioned as a contender and all prior World Bank presidents came from the political or financial sectors.

Dr. Kim is also an activist for the right to health. He began his career in global health cofounding Partners In Health (PIH) with Paul Farmer and others in 1987 with what was at the time a radical approach to community healthcare in Haiti. The PIH strategy of training community health workers to support at-home treatment for infectious diseases as well as its focus on multidrug-resistant tuberculosis were eventually adopted by WHO, which paved the way for Kim to join the organization as an adviser to the director-general in 2003. Kim became the director of WHO's HIV/AIDS department the next year. When he was nominated by President Barack Obama to serve as the next president of the World Bank in 2012, President Obama stressed the importance of Kim's development experience, declaring, "it is time for a development professional to lead the world's largest development agency."[31]

Unlike bilateral programs, the World Bank focuses on development through trade, rather than through aid. And that has led to some policies that have prioritized financial growth at the expense of health equity objectives. In the 1980s and 1990s, the World Bank had promoted point-of-service fees for healthcare.[27,32] Such fees widened health inequities, so much so that Kim declared them "unjust and unnecessary" during a speech in 2013.[33] Under Kim, the Bank heavily invested in universal health coverage and countermeasures to incentivize removing user fees, but the tension between the World Bank's mandate of economic growth and the notion of a right to health remains a delicate balancing act.

The World Bank is deeply influential in global health because it works with ministries of finance, which often have more influence over what happens in health than ministries of health themselves. The World Bank is also impactful because it is capable of backing initiative ideas with capital and loan opportunities. The World Bank financing mechanism is distinct from others within the UN system: in addition to funds from member states, the Bank also raises funds on global capital markets.[34] Its wide coffers and self-generating funding engender sustainability and flexibility. In addition to funding, the Bank also sets the tone for health economics language and metrics, including being the source of concepts such as DALYs (disability-adjusted life years), human capital, and cost-effectiveness. DALYs were put forward in a 1993 World Bank report that left an impression on Bill Gates, and the metric has since been incorporated into the Gates Foundation's own monitoring and evaluation systems, with a trickle-down impact among dozens of implementing partners.

The Bank also has a very influential network of people moving in and out of the institution, which fortifies its powerful position on the global stage. Robert McNamara resigned from serving as the US Secretary of Defense under presidents John F. Kennedy and Lyndon Johnson in 1961–1968 and was then nominated by President Johnson to become president of the World Bank. McNamara came to the Bank with a storied history, having served in the Air Force during World War II and, briefly, as the president of Ford Motor Company before accepting the appointment as secretary of defense. His military background did color his approach to economic policy, in that he believed warfare was a result of the widening income gap between nations.[35] McNamara also brought an overt sense of colonial responsibility to the World Bank, vocalizing the need for "American leadership" in organizing for development.[36] His approach at the Bank was therefore to shift focus from large infrastructure projects to poverty alleviation, including major health initiatives like family planning, and addressing onchocerciasis (river blindness). In one meeting in Washington, DC, McNamara said, "If I had my life to live over, I would concentrate all of my efforts on poverty" (Bill Foege, pers. comm., 2022).

As seen in leaders like Jim Kim and Robert McNamara, the United States is disproportionately influential in World Bank priorities; among member states, it is the largest bank shareholder.[37] The United States speaks on every issue; the president of the World Bank has always been a US citizen, and it is the only country to have individual veto power, which has been used to demand institutional policy changes, such as securing a commitment from the World Bank not to loan funds to Vietnam during the 1970s.[27,38]

Global Fund for AIDS, Tuberculosis, and Malaria

While the World Bank is the largest funder of health within the UN system, the overall largest funder of health globally is the Global Fund for AIDS, Tuberculosis, and Malaria (hereto referred to as the Global Fund).[27] It is independent from the UN system or any government, although the initial idea for the fund was put forward by UN Secretary-General Kofi Annan in April 2001. Annan called for a "war chest" of $7–10 billion annually to effectively combat HIV/AIDS and other infectious diseases.[39] Annan himself made the first contribution: he donated the $100,000 award he received for the 2001 Philadelphia Liberty Medal.[40] That summer, the UN General Assembly and the G8 endorsed the creation of the fund. It was officially founded in 2002 as a partnership of governments, civil society, technical agencies, the private sector, and people affected by HIV/AIDS, tuberculosis (TB), and malaria. It sought to accelerate efforts to end HIV/AIDS, TB, and malaria epidemics, particularly in low- and middle-income countries.

As of 2021, the Global Fund was providing 25% of all international financing for HIV programs, 77% of all international financing for TB programs, and 56% of all international financing for malaria programs.[41] The Global Fund is also the world's largest provider of overall health system–strengthening grants, providing more than $1 billion a year.[41] The Global Fund has played a key role in the COVID-19 response, allocating $4 billion to respond to COVID and to mitigate COVID's impact on HIV, TB, and malaria efforts in 2020 and 2021.[41]

The Global Fund is unique in several ways. As part of its decision not to become an implementing agency, it has no presence, offices, or staff in funding recipient countries. It also adopted a novel approach to issuing funding: recipient countries make investment decisions through a country coordinating mechanism, rather than the fund itself stipulating action items or conditions. The country coordinating mechanism is a national committee that solicits and coordinates funding requests, nominates grant recipients, and oversees program implementation, among other responsibilities. The committee itself is often broadly representative and inclusive of numerous sectors. It has representatives from academic institutions, civil society, nongovernmental organizations, government agencies, the private sector, and people living with HIV/AIDS, TB, and malaria. The approach is designed to encourage participation from various sectors within recipient countries and to be as responsive as possible to local health contexts. But the trade-off with this mechanism is that some members of the country coordinating mechanism may be direct funding recipients, creating conflicts of interest in funding allocations.

The Global Fund prides itself on its emphasis on both upward and downward accountability, meaning that it is as accountable to the people it serves as it is to its donors. As a testament to its own internal accountability, the Global Fund uncovered its own financial irregularities in four recipient countries during an investigation by internal auditors in 2011.[42]

Its funding mechanisms are designed with the explicit intention of cultivating accountability and transparency, especially through the country coordinating mechanisms. The Global Fund also implements a 15% co-financing requirement from recipient countries for each approved grant. However, developing proposals for funding that meet the technical standards expected by the Global Fund have run contrary to its mission of centering local stakeholders and decision-makers. Grant writing alone has necessitated the involvement of groups like WHO and UNICEF and has drawn in external auditors who lacked country-specific expertise and reinforced external global health decision-making.

From its inception in 2002 to September 2021, the Global Fund approved $62 billion in funding for HIV/AIDS, TB, and malaria programs in over 120 countries.[41] The Global Fund estimates its funds have saved 44 million lives and proudly boasts that the "number of deaths caused by AIDS, TB, and malaria each year has been reduced by 46% since the Global Fund was founded in 2002 in countries where the Global Fund invests."[41] Its 2021 Results Report estimates Global Fund grants have led to 21.9 million people with HIV being on antiretroviral therapy, 4.7 million people with TB being treated, and 188 million mosquito nets being distributed. Outside of these key indicators, the Global Fund's support for strengthening health systems has included things like community health worker support for malaria-prevention education in Vietnam and support to the United Nations Development Programme's solar panel program for warehouses that store and distribute temperature-controlled pharmaceuticals in Zambia.[43,44]

But it hasn't all been rosy. As a result of COVID-19-related disruptions, key programmatic indicators for the Global Fund went down in 2021 for the first time since its founding. Malaria was the least impacted, but the number of tests among suspected case-patients still dropped by 4.3%. Related to TB, about 1 million fewer people with TB were treated in 2020 compared to 2019, and the number of people treated for drug-resistant TB in recipient countries dropped by 19%. For HIV, the number of people reached with HIV-prevention programs and services declined by 11% and the number of HIV tests taken declined by 22%.[41]

The largest share of the Global Fund dollars are for HIV (about 42.5%), followed by malaria (29.5%), TB (15.3%), and TB/HIV (10%). A smaller portion of funding, to the tune of about $1.5 billion, is also allocated to health systems strengthening and multicomponent funding.[45] Even though the allocations for health system strengthening are small compared to its disease-specific allocations, the

Global Fund is still the world's largest provider of grants to strengthen overall health systems.

Early on, the Global Fund realized the need to address the broader health systems within a given context and its impact on its three focus epidemics.[46] The lack of physical health facilities and trained health workers, weak procurements systems, and poor health information systems were clear impediments to control of HIV, TB, and malaria.[47] Evaluations in the 2007 and 2008 rollout of antiretroviral treatment in Zambia and South Africa demonstrated that a focus on disease-specific efforts was exacerbating the fractures within strained national health systems.[48,49] The few trained health workers who existed were seeking out programs funded by the Global Fund rather than public sector programs because Global Fund programs were considered more desirable employers, given their higher salaries and greater opportunities for advancement. Of course, these challenges were not unique to the Global Fund, but they were particularly pronounced in Global Fund programs given their size. In response to these outcomes, the Global Fund began setting aside funding for health systems strengthening and introduced a requirement that funding proposals demonstrate how the proposed activities would complement existing health plans, strategies, and activities.[50]

Today, public sector contributions make up 95% of all Global Fund financing. The United States is the single largest donor—congressional appropriations in 2001–2022 constituted nearly $23 billion or over a third of the Global Fund's total funding since 2001.[45] The $23 billion does not include a one-time allocation of $3.5 billion in 2021 specifically for the COVID response.[45] To put that amount in context, the regular US appropriations for that year were less than half that amount ($1.6 billion) and that single donation accounts for about 6% of the Global Fund's financing—ever. As with the World Bank, the United States has an outsized influence on the Global Fund. The United States has its own permanent seat on the board and sits on the board's Ethics & Governance Committee and the Strategy Committee, giving it a central role in Global Fund governance and oversight.

Funding from the United States is generally initiated by the US president, who makes requests for funding. Congress then makes the final decision on allocations through PEPFAR (see chapter 7), often matching what the president requests or even increasing the allocation. For example, former President Trump suggested cuts to Global Fund allocations, which Congress rejected. Congress's significant financial support over the last two decades has been accompanied by some restrictions, including requiring that US contributions not exceed 33% of total contributions from all donors—which was invoked during FY 2004.

But not all financing is from governments. The largest private sector donor to the Global Fund is Red—better recognized as "(RED)." Many remember the star-studded Gap campaign from the late 2000s, where ad participants sported T-shirts emblazoned with slogans like "assu(red)," "empowe(red)," or "admi(red)," or the red iPhones and iPods. The (RED) concept was founded in 2006 by U2 star Bono and Bobby Shriver and sought to raise awareness and funds to help eliminate HIV/AIDS in eight African nations. All (RED) proceeds went to the Global Fund. As of September 2020, (RED) had generated over $650 million to support Global Fund grants.[51]

(RED) is an interesting case study for the role of the private sector in global health. It raised immense social awareness of the HIV/AIDS epidemic in the African continent through its extensive marketing campaign, and it rallied support from large companies that are not commonly players in global health. To name a small selection of involved companies: American Express launched a dedicated credit card, Giorgio Armani created a clothing line, Motorola offered special edition cell phones, Canon ran a special release of its SD990 camera, Hallmark produced greeting cards, The Killers donated the proceeds from their annual Christmas song release, and the Belvedere vodka company produced (RED) bottles. But critics have questioned the value of the advertising price tag and whether or not the extensive advertising efforts really yielded a result proportional to the investment. Some accused the companies of profiting off "cause branding," or using diseases as a marketing strategy, spending millions in advertising that could have gone directly to the cause.

That being said, it is unlikely many of these companies would have otherwise engaged in direct contributions. This approach has mobilized a slew of companies to participate in fundraising to address global health issues, ultimately covering 2% of the Global Fund budget. Two percent may not sound like much, but one official at the fund has noted that this influx of funding has supported programs in 136 countries. (RED) itself does not advertise—companies pay (RED) to label their products with the brand, cover the advertising budget themselves, and then donate a portion of sales to the fund. (RED) sets forth a promising example of how advocates can work with the private sector to mobilize critical funding for global health.

Broadly, what the Global Fund does well is unite public and private donors under one very independent multilateral financing entity. As a testament to the Global Fund's neutrality, the entity was founded under notoriously neutral Swiss law. Its sheer size is remarkably impactful: having given $62 billion over 20 years has left a heavy footprint. But the COVID-19 pandemic erased a number of hard-fought gains in HIV, TB, and malaria, and called into question the role of the Global Fund in pandemic preparedness and global health security generally. And even given the Global Fund's impressive record, its budget is still just a small portion of the estimated resources needed to reach ambitious disease-eradication targets.

Multilateralism in Action: Access to COVID-19 Tools Accelerator (ACT-Accelerator)

The COVID-19 pandemic sparked a flurry of development for new diagnostic tests, treatments, and vaccines. In 2020 alone, the FDA approved over 300 test and collection kits, WHO was tracking over 1,700 clinical trials for promising treatments, and 321 vaccine candidates were undergoing testing.[52-54] The Access to COVID-19 Tools Accelerator—or the ACT-Accelerator—sought to end the acute phase of the COVID-19 pandemic by accelerating the development and production of, and equitable access to, the resulting tests, treatments, and vaccines.[55]

The ACT-Accelerator is multilateralism in action, designed to use its size and connections as leverage for global benefit. It is not a decision-making body or a new organization, but instead describes itself as a framework for collaboration. This framework is jointly led by the Global Fund, the World Bank, WHO, Gavi, the Foundation for Innovative New Diagnostics (FIND), the Coalition for Epidemic Preparedness Innovations (CEPI), UNICEF, the Wellcome Trust, the Bill & Melinda Gates Foundation, and Unitaid. ACT-Accelerator is organized into four pillars: diagnostics, therapeutics, vaccines (aka the COVAX Facility), and the health systems and response connector.

For high-income countries, the COVAX Facility was essentially an insurance policy while vaccines were still undergoing clinical trials and their efficacy and success rates were unknown. The facility offered a large and diverse portfolio of vaccine candidates and served as an alternative to more risky bilateral agreements between a given government and a vaccine manufacturer. But for low-income countries, it was often their only hope of securing COVID-19 vaccines, as bidding in the open market was unaffordable for 92 countries. As such, the COVAX Facility sought to be a vehicle for ensuring equitable distribution of safe and effective vaccines by using investments from high- and middle-income countries to subsidize the cost of doses to low-income countries. The COVAX Facility pledged to make 100 million doses available by March 2021, 600 million doses by the end of July 2021, and 2 billion doses by the end of 2021.

That did not pan out as intended. Most high-income countries pursued their own bilateral agreements with vaccine manufacturers, quickly procured most of the world's stock, and then donated funds to the COVAX Facility for purchasing doses for poorer nations. Before vaccines even reached shelves, 32 high-income countries representing 13% of the global population had purchased half the estimated 2021 production capacity.[56] Canada alone pre-purchased nine doses per citizen.[56] Though Canada did ultimately donate its excess, their over-order approach demonstrates the mentality of many high-income countries at the time: purchase in excess and only once national demand was met, share beyond their borders.[57]

In January 2021, WHO Director-General Tedros Adhanom Ghebreyesus accused the world of being on the brink of a "catastrophic moral failure" driven by a "vaccine apartheid," noting that while one in four people in high-income countries had received at least one vaccine, the same ratio was one in 500 people in low-income nations.[58–60] This vaccine nationalism, combined with supply bottlenecks, gravely hampered the COVAX Facility's ability to meet its goals, providing only 175 million doses by August or only about 29% of its original target.[61]

While the COVAX Facility failed to meet its original targets, it was the best and only global mechanism for COVID vaccine procurement among low-income nations. Through its size and backing from CEPI and UNICEF, the COVAX Facility did succeed in making *billions* of doses available to countries that could not have otherwise competed in the open market. Multilateralism was not efficient in its pursuit of vaccine equity, hampered principally by vaccine nationalism, but it was a critical counterbalance to hoarding and chaotic procurement.

As COVID cases have declined and public attention has waned, the ACT-Accelerator has struggled to secure continued funding. Though the framework for collaboration was never intended to be a permanent fixture, the need for continued coordinated efforts persists. As of July 2022, only 20% of the population in the African continent was fully vaccinated.[62] The potential closure of the ACT-Accelerator raises questions about how the global community will continue to fund the fight against COVID, and particularly, how lower-income countries will secure adequate supplies of vaccines, diagnostics, and treatments. There *is*, however, broad recognition that any subsequent effort will require multilateral coordination.

UNICEF

The Beginning of UNICEF

In an attempt to flee the Nazi onslaught, in late 1939, more than 1 million people fled Poland; nearly 100,000 of those arrived north of Iran. The British authorities helped the refugees through a new organization, the Middle East Relief and Refugee Administration (MERRA). The organization counted 999 orphans in the settlement.

By 1944, the organization handed responsibilities to the United Nations Relief and Rehabilitation Administration (UNRRA). The prime minister of New Zealand, Peter Fraser, arranged for all 999 children to live out their futures in New Zealand.

According to Maggie Black, in her book on the history of UNICEF:

> About a year later, Mr. Wladyslaw Gomulka, who was then Vice-Premier of Poland, complained good-naturedly that UNRRA had "stolen" some of his children, but UNRRA's reputation in Poland was remarkable—"To us, UNRRA is a holy word"—and he quickly agreed that they could not have gone to a better country.[63]

With UNRRA's founding in 1943 to help children, displaced persons, and survivors of concentrations camps, that story quickly became one of its greatest successes. However, despite its good intentions, delegates from the United States feared that broadcasting those good intentions would not be well-received by the public. The delegates feared the public would perceive UNRRA as "taking bread out of American mouths."[63]

Even though Winston Churchill was a leading contributor to the founding of UNRRA, after two years of operation, he became a critic. The assistance that UNRRA was providing was largely contributed by the United States and Western allies, and then largely allocated to socialist countries in eastern Europe. On March 6, 1946, Churchill delivered his "Iron Curtain"* speech in Fulton, Missouri.

> From what I have seen of our Russian friends and Allies during the war, I am convinced that there is nothing they admire so much as strength, and there is nothing for which they have less respect than for weakness, especially military weakness. . . . We cannot afford, if we can help it, to work on narrow margins, offering temptations to a trial of strength.[64]

Such criticism—plus political and military distrust—ultimately threatened the continuation of UNRRA. However, its staff advocated

---

* Churchill did not originate this phrase. Joseph Goebbels first used it in a speech in late 1944 and in an article published in the *London Times* in early 1945.

for a permanent organization to continue aid to children. Thus was born the United Nations International Children's Emergency Fund (UNICEF), established on December 11, 1946. According to Maggie Black, "The word 'emergency' was of vital importance in securing the support of some governments that were not keen to see any new institution which resembled even part of UNRRA's work."[63,65]

Maurice Pate was the first executive director of UNICEF. While Pate thought his position would be temporary, as the organization was addressing postwar emergencies, he quickly saw the need to extend UNICEF's life span. He believed it was a moral duty for everyone to give a helping hand to those less fortunate.

The Jim Grant Era

UNICEF has a glorious history, which hit a high point when Jim Grant, a lawyer, became its executive director. Typically, when someone asks you to pass the salt at a banquet, it is not meant as a segue for a question about child development and survival. Unless you were Jim Grant. As the executive director at UNICEF, during banquets with presidents or prime ministers, he would ask them to pass the salt. Then, he would take a dropper of liquid from his pocket and dispense a drop or two onto the salt. If it turned blue, the salt was iodized. If it did not turn blue, Grant would go into his speech about how the absence of iodine in a critical point in development left many children mentally compromised. He would then talk about several other simple interventions that could pay huge dividends.[66]

Jim Grant advocated for what was termed GOBI (Growth charts, Oral rehydration, Breastfeeding, and Immunization). He unveiled plans to make these four low-cost techniques available to almost every child in every developing country. His plan resulted in some labeling him the "mad American."

At that time, UNICEF only had projects that reached thousands of children, but Grant hoped to reach up to 500 million children. Despite the skeptics, the four low-cost interventions were ushered in with the Child Survival and Development Revolution of the 1980s. GOBI became part of the global health vocabulary.

As Jon Rohde phrased it in a UNICEF publication on this great leader,

> Jim constantly reminded us that the true state of a society is measured by the state of its poor, not by averages. . . . Jim's view was that inequality and relative poverty would be the great challenges of the future, but that the great task of the present was to defeat absolute poverty—to put a safety net below which no one on earth should be allowed to fall. This is what bred Jim's preoccupation with "survival"—surely not all there is to life, but an essential and inalienable first right.[66]

Grant made incredible strides with the Child Survival and Development Revolution. Whenever meeting with presidents and prime ministers, Grant would know their country's immunization rates, oral rehydration and salt usage, as well as the mortality rates for children under five years of age. In his mind, there were no excuses to not adopt these four interventions.

Upon asking for an immunization level progress report in El Salvador, Grant was not satisfied with the representative's response that the levels were not rising due to the war. "Well, why don't they stop the war so they can immunize the kids?" he asked[66] (Bill Foege, pers. comm, 2022). Subsequently, Grant traveled to El Salvador, where the UNICEF staff partnered with the Catholic church to negotiate with the government and guerilla leaders. Three separate days of every year until the war ended were under cease-fire to enable children's immunization. This was not the only instance in which Grant negotiated the halting of war for the sake of the children. Nils Thedin first formulated the concept of "children as a zone of peace" in 1983. Grant showed its promise. Grant was involved in negotiations to halt war in Lebanon in 1987, Sudan in 1989, and Iraq in 1991[66] (Bill Foege, pers. comm., 2022).

Eventually, GOBI transitioned to GOBI-FFF to include family planning, female education, and food security. But it was still a program focused on high-priority interventions, rather than on building infrastructures.

When a new executive director of UNICEF stepped in, immunization coverage and ORT (oral rehydration therapy) use decreased. Grant's leadership and vision are often cited as the driving force behind the success of the Child Survival and Development Revolution. But ironically, this vision was not even emulated in UNICEF after his death.

Nearly eight decades later, the fear of "taking bread out of American mouths" is still held as a criticism of global health development and foreign assistance.

Concluding Thoughts
BILL FOEGE

Multilateral organizations are part of the evolutionary progress of global health. In general, they are more robust than bilateral organizations because more groups are invested in the outcomes. But they also present challenges in execution because of the turnover of key personnel and the increased chance of internal conflict.

Jim Grant's insistence that eliminating poverty should be our ultimate future goal prompts a comment on famine. At the present time, *the only reason children starve is because of war, conflicts, or political barriers*. Food and transportation are sufficient to solve any famine in the absence of those problems.

Another aspect of global health evolution is that in addition to changes in personnel, institutions change. The World Bank, for example, formed to provide economic assistance to poor countries and to speed up development, ironically has become the largest contributor to health financing in the UN system and second only to the Global Fund in the field of global health. The World Bank has incredible influence because it works with ministers of finance rather than ministers of health. It also commonly sets the tone for health economics and metrics language, including DALYs (disability-adjusted life years), human capital, cost-effectiveness, and the like. It has a very influential network of people moving in and out of the bank. And recently, as stated, it even had a president, Dr. Jim Kim, who was a global health worker.

The triumph of multilateral agencies is the example they set of donor countries working together rather than each presenting a different scenario to recipient countries. At their best, organizations such as the Global Fund and Gavi consolidate rather than fractionate health assistance. Their existence is particularly useful when agencies such as WHO see them as partners rather than competitors.

The potential dark side was demonstrated by Dr. Hiroshi Nakajima, who regarded all health activities as the domain of WHO and made cooperation very difficult. The fact that this has happened should be a sign it could happen again. Any restructuring of WHO should guard against that possibility.

The proliferation of agencies presents challenges for recipient countries, but it also increases the number of people participating in global health. While bilateral agencies are attractive to donating countries, in practice such agencies still have to coordinate with countries and multilateral programs. This is a clear difference from the colonial age, when stand-alone programs were common. Likewise, as will be seen in the following chapter on nongovernmental organizations, the numbers have increased dramatically, but to be successful they, too, must coordinate with countries as well as multilateral programs. Efficiency would suggest tighter rules of coordination, but practicality thrives on people of passion pursuing a specific disease or subsegment of global health, and often they receive funding from bilateral and multilateral organizations.

CHAPTER 9

The Rise of NGOs

KIERA CHAN

Consider three scenarios, all in different points in history across the world, but with one thing in common. In 1945 during World War II in Holland, a girl, hungry and cold, receives a package full of canned food, powdered milk, coffee, and material for clothes.[1] The girl rushes home, her face alight with joy and hope. The young girl is Audrey Hepburn, and the package is a "CARE package." In 1987, protestors crowd Wall Street in the United States in the midst of the AIDS crisis, fighting for affordable prices for a lifesaving drug.[2] In 2015, a refugee camp, complete with tents and bustling makeshift streets, sprawls out for miles and miles. This is one of the world's largest camps, Dadaab, the size of some of the biggest cities in Kenya.[3] Volunteers, workers, and camp coordinators work together to keep the camp running and will be ready at a moment's notice to respond to the next crisis.

All three of these scenarios are linked by one common facet: the lifesaving work, coordination, and resources brought by nongovernmental organizations (NGOs). These scenarios represent the vast history and diversity of NGO work, as well as the complexity of their role in global health.

What Is an NGO?

An NGO is any nonstate citizens' group targeted on a specific issue and structured around a common mission.[4] Founded by citizens themselves, NGOs can be for profit, not for profit, private, public, religiously affiliated, or not religious. This type of group is founded by citizens themselves, independent of any government influence. NGOs are becoming an increasingly common method of global health service delivery and have become the "favored child" of governments and public health leaders in development contexts because of their close connection with the community and their relatively low-budget ventures compared to many government or private responses.[5] NGOs can range in size from a small group to a large, complex organization with annual revenues of over $1 billion. NGOs can have diverse interests, goals, and backgrounds.[6] For example, some like Orbis International, are focused on one disease; others, such as Partners In Health, alleviate poverty through an array of community-based measures.[7] NGOs have been sought out as the desired medium of global health program implementation because of their effectiveness on the ground.

Today, NGOs have become the third sector, representing a wide variety of public interests and voluntary work.[8] This contrasts with the public sector, which is the state, and the private sector, which is the business or for-profit sector. Separate from these two sectors, NGOs often have the freedom to act in innovative ways, while also modifying their strategies to become more efficient and sustainable because of their limited funding. The third sector now performs many of the functions that the public sector performs or was supposed to perform, such as providing basic health services for low-income communities. Thus, NGOs often receive funding from the public sector to achieve these tasks. The NGO sector often represents the needs of citizens themselves, which is often how NGOs are legitimized in the economy.

In 1940, only about 427 NGOs existed in the United States.[9] Now, there are an estimated 10 million worldwide.[8] They include emergency relief organizations such as CARE International, human rights organizations such as Amnesty International, and health-related organizations such as Doctors Without Borders. Their missions and scopes are varied. Indeed, there is now an organization for almost any cause imaginable.

The term "nongovernmental organization" was coined in 1950 by the United Nations to differentiate between private organizations and intergovernmental organizations.[6] Since then, NGOs have been legitimized and recognized as entities that can work in partnership with bilateral agencies and international governmental bodies such as the UN. Ever since the dawn of the UN in 1945, it has included NGOs in its decision-making.[10] NGOs are granted partnership and voice within the UN system via the Economic and Social Council (ECOSOC), where they can participate in advancing sustainable development. NGOs can apply for consultative status through the UN so that they can engage in commissions and programs to help translate development goals into actual change within the lives of their beneficiaries. NGOs participate in conferences and build valuable partnerships with the UN bodies, giving constructive feedback for policymaking and participating in policy implementation. Since the conception of the ECOSOC Resolution, which governs the partnership between NGOs and the UN, the number of participating NGOs has risen from 41 to over 5,000 organizations.

The First NGOs

In 1830, Alexis de Tocqueville, a French diplomat and political philosopher, wrote in awe how devoted American citizens were to civil society.[9] He noted in his treatise *Democracy in America* that Americans of all different backgrounds and conditions were joining together to form voluntary associations to solve any problem. This form of philanthropy was at the heart of American democracy. The American philanthropic voluntary community has become the largest in the world, with unprecedented numbers of NGOs and amounts of private giving from the American public.

The Red Cross Movement, founded in 1863 by Henri Dunant, was an important step in the long line of humanitarian organizations that would soon follow.[11] Dunant witnessed the horrors of the Battle of Solferino in the Second Battle for Italian Independence and proposed a partnership of national relief societies to alleviate suffering during the war and provide the much-needed care that was absent during his time. His ideas to develop a committee of relief and an internationally recognized agreement to address care to the war-wounded led to the creation of the International Committee of the Red Cross (ICRC) and the original Geneva Convention. The ICRC urged governments to adopt the convention so that militaries had to agree to care for wounded soldiers regardless of what side they were on. The Red Cross Movement grew, and after World War I, the League of Red Cross Societies was formed. Now, the International Red Cross Movement is the largest humanitarian network in the world. It includes the ICRC, the International Federation of the Red Cross and Red Crescent Societies, and 190 National Societies.[12] ICRC is not an NGO—it is a private organization. Yet the creation of the Red Cross movement set the stage for NGOs, particularly relief organizations that were impartial to politics or war.

The Second Industrial Revolution: ALA

The period of the second industrial revolution, from the 1870s to World War I, brought a slow and steady rise of NGOs as well as a new commitment to human rights.[5] The establishment of the Income Tax Law in 1917 permitted American citizens to deduct up to 15% of their taxable income for charitable contributions—formally marking the beginning of an era of charitable giving. Although the Income Tax Amendment looks much different today, individuals can still deduct charitable contributions on their taxes. During this era, faith-based organizations started to spread across the globe, stemming from the Catholic and Protestant churches.[13] The number of NGOs was still low during this time but would soon face new changes in the 21st century.

The second industrial revolution was marked by urban overcrowding and poor hygiene, leading to a rise in infectious diseases. The rise in tuberculosis gave birth to the American Lung Association (ALA) in

Chicago, one of the first public health NGOs in the United States.[14] In 1904, the National Association for the Study and Prevention of Tuberculosis was created to support a small patient-treatment facility. The association's goal was to create free clinics for treating tuberculosis in every city and county.

The mission started out as a small operation to raise money for the treatment facility, a tiny sanitorium in Delaware. One of the doctors at the clinic asked his cousin, Emily Bissell, to raise $300, which was needed to keep the facility open. She proceeded to design Christmas seals, small stickers to put on envelopes with holiday messages. These were America's first Christmas seals, which generated much support from the public, raising over $3,000. The organization funded research, which led to advances in the X-ray and skin test, soon to become the gold standard diagnostic tests for tuberculosis. The organization successfully reduced the incidence of tuberculosis and soon expanded into the ALA, which targeted other pulmonary diseases as well. The Christmas seal still represents the power of volunteerism and public support among Americans today. Even into the 21st century, ALA remains driven toward its mission to improve lung disease and increase research toward preventing lung disease.

NGOs after World War II

CARE

After World War II, new development and humanitarian goals emerged, spurring the formation of larger NGOs. Although NGOs such as the Red Cross existed before the two world wars, they did not spring up with such force until after World War II.[5]

One such NGO was CARE, one of the oldest and largest NGOs in the United States; many others were created after World War II.[1] When Germany was left in ruins by years of war, and many people suffered from lack of food, the Marshall Plan was signed into action to help rebuild Europe through economic development.[15] This marked the start of the modern-day concept of international development aid.

Many NGOs were enlisted to help reconstruct Europe with the help of the US military at this time. President Roosevelt specifically created a War Relief Control Board to oversee the efforts of these NGOs.[16]

Created largely at the insistence of the War Relief Control Board, CARE was developed to fill a niche for an individual-to-individual package service that other relief agencies were not equipped to handle. The military was in charge of providing supplies such as food after the war. However, the board jumped at the chance to transfer this responsibility to another organization, helping to organize a purchase deal of food packages for the organization. CARE purchased from the US Army 2.8 million 10-in-1 rations, so named because they were initially designed to feed 10 men for a single day or a single man for 10 days.

CARE first started in 1945 as a one-shot program designed to deliver packages of food to World War II survivors in Europe. The idea was borne out of a food distribution service inspired by Herbert Hoover's American Relief Administration's plan during World War I. The Cooperative League of USA raised over $100,000 to aid with the rehabilitation efforts after World War II and decided to set up a non-profit cooperative run by various member organizations interested in the food aid system. Unlike most humanitarian organizations at the time, CARE ensured that donors could feel that they truly made a difference by allowing them to send a package directly to a recipient. The donor was notified when the package was received; the recipient was assured that the package was given by a compassionate American individual. The name CARE was thought of by the wife of Lincoln Park, one of CARE's founders. He explained to her that American donors could pay $10 to send a voucher to a recipient in Europe to pick up a CARE package. She came up with the name of "Cooperative for American Remittances to Europe."

Although these packages had several flaws—they contained cigarettes, for example, which were not yet widely viewed as dangerous to one's health—they allowed the organization to send direct aid immediately to those in need. In 1948, CARE reported that it supplied recipients with $52 million worth of food. The operation grew bigger than it ever could have imagined, and donors soon started sending money to send a package to anyone, instead of a specific person. The organization was not designed for this, so the board initially wanted to send those checks back to the donors. However, the organization soon evolved to send general aid to anyone. In 1948, during the Berlin Blockade, CARE airlifted over 200,000 packages to Western Berlin. At the time, a raisin-growing cooperative in California had a large surplus of raisins so it donated them to CARE. One result: Berliners who received CARE packages during the Soviet blockade called the airplanes "Roisenbomber." In 1953, CARE's operations started moving into other parts of the world, and its name changed to "Cooperative for American Relief Everywhere." In 1955, CARE considered dissolving, as most of its European missions closed and the war recovery program was complete, but the organization chose to scale back its missions instead.

UNHCR

Other institutions were established before and during World War II with the help of NGOs worldwide. The United Nations High Commissioner for Refugees, or UNHCR, was established in 1950 with the aim to help European refugees.[17]

Before it was created, NGOs were massively overwhelmed with the influx of refugees spurred by the Balkan Wars in 1912, the Russian Revolution and the failed counterrevolution in 1917, and the fall of the Ottoman Empire. Led by the ICRC, NGOs urged the League of Nations in 1921 to create an agency to coordinate the aid needed for European refugees. Thus, the League appointed its first High Commissioner for Refugees, Norwegian Fridtjof Nansen.[18] After World War II, the mandate of the commissioner was expanded, and the UNHCR was formally established by the UN along with over 30 NGOs. The UNHCR was only meant to serve the short-term needs of the European refugees; however, it soon grew to become one of the main implementing partners among refugee crises globally.

NGOs and the Cold War

After World War II, the baby boom generation in the United States brought new prosperity to America, triggering the formation of more NGOs. Increased prosperity brought in more donations, nonprofits, and volunteerism. The decolonization and independence of African states during the 1960s and 1970s brought NGO attention to development aid in Africa and emphasized the role of NGO aid in the peace movement.[19] During the Cold War, the United States and the Soviet Union were strengthening their military systems and stockpiling arms. Meanwhile, NGOs were left to deal with civil society issues as well as humanitarian work in low-income countries.[13]

The 21st century and the post–Cold War era created a perfect storm of conditions that allowed NGOs to emerge at unprecedented levels.[20] At the end of the Cold War, a new policy agenda established a mindset of liberal economics that reduced the role of the government in the US economy and prompted the role of NGO work as a means of democracy. Under this new liberal economic theory, governments were expected to create an enabling environment for private sector initiatives in the economy. This also meant that social services were distributed through privatization, often leaving NGOs to take over these activities.

The end of the Cold War also led to a decrease in aid to gain foreign allies. At that time, low-income countries were experiencing a decline in public and financial support of their governments, which led to significant deteriorations of their market economies. The occurrence of weak states and markets left no choice but for NGOs to move in to provide aid. During the Cold War, communist nations withdrew from the International Monetary Fund.[21] The fund and the World Bank also started to cut funds due to globalization, which prompted more NGOs to provide assistance. The World Bank not only encouraged the presence of NGOs in international assistance but also funded NGOs to work with local governments. The World Bank and other donors such as the US Agency for International Development (USAID) started funding NGOs more heavily because they believed that governments were too centralized at the time.

The rise of NGOs was legitimized during the Cold War as they became increasingly professionalized and supported by donors and development partners.[22] More NGOs were also founded outside of the United States at this time. During the Cold War, a divide between the West, the socialist, and the resource-poor countries grew. USAID declared that a "vibrant civil society is an essential component of a democratic polity" and "that the Agency will concentrate its support for civil society on . . . nongovernmental organizations." Soon, the term "civil society" was equated with NGOs. As the Cold War was ending, USAID was experiencing budget cuts because the US Government was cutting foreign aid funds. With less funding, USAID had to fund low-cost operations such as NGOs. Additionally, the Cold War showed institutions such as USAID and the World Bank that states were possibly corrupt, which led to increased financing from USAID for NGOs.[6]

During the Cold War, power vacuums caused African states such as those in sub-Saharan Africa to become even weaker and susceptible to corruption due to years of colonialization and Western control during the war.[21] The structural adjustment programs—economic policies for developing countries implemented by the International Monetary Fund—exacerbated economic conditions, even though they were meant to stimulate economic growth. NGOs often filled the gap and provided basic social services that the states could not provide.[23] Most donors preferred funding NGOs instead of channeling development assistance through governments. Donors also saw NGOs as more efficient and able to provide services with very little funds. This preference for providing NGOs with funding, instead of states or governmental organizations, was most likely caused by the inefficiencies of many bilateral and federal agencies.[5]

Doctors Without Borders

The period of the 1960s and 1970s—with decolonization of African states, civil wars, and conflict after colonialism—gave birth to the modern humanitarianism and NGO work we see today.[9] One example was the Nigerian Civil War, or the Biafran War, which advanced the role of NGOs in humanitarianism and public health and also established what the "Third World" was and how "Western intervention" could take place.[24] After Nigeria's independence from Britain in 1960, the remnants of colonial rule and the creation of territorial borders that reflected ethnic groups created a religious and ethnic divide in the country, causing conflict over political dominance.[25] In 1966, the conflict escalated, and the United Kingdom, fearing it would lose dominance in Nigeria, dispatched arms, and war broke out. The United Kingdom became involved because of the Biafran territory's oil supply. And this war, unlike some of the others in Africa at the same time, caught the West's attention for the same reason.

During the Nigerian Civil War, France provided volunteer doctors to work under the ICRC in Biafra. These doctors were so impacted by the horror of war[26] that, after the war ended, they formed a group called Médicins Sans Frontières (or Doctors Without Borders, in English). This group spoke out against bad policies, saying priority should always be given to the health and well-being of people.

Thus, Doctors Without Borders established a new type of humanitarianism, revolutionary for its time. Unlike most NGOs, it argued that the welfare of the people far outweighs any border, nation, religion, or political affiliation. Although most NGOs prided themselves on being neutral, nonsectarian, and not affiliated with any government or donors, sometimes this feature of neutrality interfered with an NGO's ability to carry out its missions. Doctors Without Borders' main concept was called *témoignage* or "to witness." This NGO believed that it should act as witness to the people it served and speak out against human rights violations in response. To remain completely independent, it decided to rely on individual donors for funding, refusing funds from any corporation or government. This allowed the organization to distribute aid without furthering any political or institutional agenda. Doctors Without Borders is a key example of how many NGOs were created during this time and gained popular support through their work in controversial settings such as the Biafran War. It was no coincidence that France was also undergoing social changes with the protests of 1968, which started a peace movement and political turmoil.

Doctors Without Borders has since provided medical assistance and emergency care in over 80 countries and has treated over 100 million patients. It frequently denounces human rights violations. For example, in 2014, it increased its activities in the Central African Republic to respond to violence. Although the French government itself had declared that the conflict had subsided, Doctors Without Borders spoke out against the international community and government and raised awareness about the escalating violence and human rights violations. This NGO asserted that, above all, the health of the people should come first, regardless of a state's invitation to serve in its country. Thus, it often crosses into borders surreptitiously to provide care, ignoring the standard NGO commitment toward noninterference. This has led to trouble with some governments. For instance, in 1984, Doctors Without Borders was working in Ethiopia to respond to famine crises when the government forcefully relocated millions, causing much suffering and death. This NGO spoke out against the government and was promptly expelled from the country. Despite these incidents, the organization remains devoted to its mission of morality and care for citizens, no matter how involved it must become in conflict or politics.

The Golden Era of Global Health

Social upheavals in the 1970s and 1980s brought attention to new political, social, and human rights issues, prompting more NGOs to be formed. The increase in mass higher education and urbanization has fueled the rise of NGOs today.[7]

Technology has also made the proliferation of NGOs easier than ever before. It facilitated the rise in communication and telecommunication methods. Lower cost and higher-quality technologies allowed NGOs to spread their missions across the globe and to collaborate and advocate in ways so that even smaller, low-budget organizations could participate in global health.[8] During the AIDS epidemic, funding for global health skyrocketed, and transnational advocacy permitted the distribution of low-cost, generic treatments for those in need. The 1990s were known as a "golden era" for NGOs.[22] Compared to the previous decade, NGOs in one country alone would double during this era. Furthermore, the AIDS epidemic in the 1980s and 1990s, along with other public health crises, ushered in a new commitment toward global health.

The AIDS epidemic helped to bring light to some of the work NGOs brought to the arena of global health and helped the rise of more public health NGOs.[27] Not only did NGOs help set trends in institutionalized interventions for AIDS, but also donors and governments finally recognized the power of NGOs, which soon led to their becoming the "favored child" of development.[5] NGOs were often among the first to respond, providing communities with counseling, healthcare, and other modes of support. Because NGOs were smaller and less bureaucratic, they could provide services almost immediately.[28] Some NGOs, such as Doctors Without Borders, also went unhindered by politics that acted as barriers for governmental institutions to provide services and information around sensitive subjects such as condom use. NGOs' community-based nature also aided in targeting and transforming community attitudes and behaviors from the inside out. Unlike bigger institutions, NGOs were also adept at reaching the most marginalized and vulnerable populations, such as sex workers, who might be hesitant to reach out to more mainstream healthcare services.[29]

AIDS Epidemic-Associated NGOs

NGO WORK IN UGANDA

The success story of Uganda is one that is paraded as a poster child for intervention methods for AIDS. With the decline of infection from 30% in the 1990s to 10% in just under a decade, Uganda represents one of the world's most compelling cases for a dramatic decline in HIV/AIDS.[30] Although some of this success can be attributed to the government's commitment toward making HIV/AIDS a national political issue, most was due to the role of NGOs in the epidemic, thanks to coordination from the Ugandan government. The first case was detected in 1982; by the middle of the 1980s, the country had a full-blown epidemic.

The government established an AIDS Control Programme in 1986, starting a rigorous governmental campaign to mobilize political, community, and institutional actors across the country toward fighting AIDS. This government action on AIDS can be traced to Dr. Seth Berkley, who was working for the Task Force for Child Survival in Uganda. He showed the Ugandan president data on the alarming rise of HIV in pregnant women. The president's response was, basically, "If *I* know this, *everyone* should," and published Berkley's graph in the newspaper (Bill Foege, pers. comm., 2023).

This coordination and centralization of public health action helped to legitimize the work of NGOs in the community and soon gave rise to a large cohort of NGOs aimed at targeting AIDS within the country.[31] By 2003, an estimated 2,500 NGOs were working on HIV/AIDS in increasing numbers. Furthermore, the government's authority helped to minimize conflicts or duplication between competing NGOs.

The rise in NGOs in the 1970s and 1980s increased during the 1990s due to the growing need for support for the rising number of orphans and those ostracized due to HIV/AIDS.[32] At first, these NGOs were merely informal gatherings of small support groups; however, they soon grew to become one of the world's largest networks of NGOs aimed at fighting a single cause. The donor community's preference toward NGOs globally stemmed from a lack of confidence in the government's ability to manage the AIDS crisis. This, together with the recognition that NGOs could effectively mobilize the community and address issues of stigmatization, led to increasing acceptance of NGO work by development agencies and the public. The World Health Organization (WHO) Global Programme on AIDS in 1980 soon legitimized NGO work in several international networks, such as the International Council of AIDS Service Organizations.[33]

One such NGO was The AIDS Support Organization (TASO) in Uganda, established in 1987 to address the support needs for those impacted by HIV/AIDS.[28] The founder, Noerine Kaleeba, recognized the need for an organization consisting of the people affected by the virus, when her husband suffered discrimination and inferior treatment before dying at a hospital. Most of the trained volunteers and workers were themselves infected with HIV or had lost a loved one from the virus, which increased local resource mobilization and increased democratic governance. TASO soon grew to become the largest NGO support organization in Africa.[34] The Ugandan government itself requested TASO to set up clinics for patients with HIV/AIDS. Hospitals across the country sought out TASO's expertise in training for their own doctors and medical staff. WHO and the Joint United Nations Programme on HIV/AIDS insisted that TASO increase its reach and soon funded the delivery of antiretroviral therapy for its beneficiaries. TASO not only improved the quality of life for those affected by the virus, but it also reduced the rate of transmission and provided hope to those infected.

TASO and the thousands of other NGOs in Uganda bridged relationships between community members, generated awareness, and provided funding from the international community for HIV/AIDS programs.[35] Specifically, NGOs were able to promote behavioral change programs such as those aimed at decreasing multiple sexual partners. The involvement of religious organizations, in particular, led to active participation of communities in reducing the spread of HIV/AIDS, as faith-based organizations are extremely influential in Uganda. Women's organizations also contributed toward the action with their "zero grazing" strategies, aimed at men engaged in multiple sexual relationships. These programs were targeted at older men with disposable income, believed to be the core transmitters of the epidemic. Now, Uganda is used as a global reference point for the effectiveness of such NGO programs in the decline of AIDS.

FAITH-BASED NGOS

The role of faith-based NGOs in the AIDS epidemic cannot be overestimated. In general, religious NGOs provide significant amounts of healthcare in Africa and demonstrate their crucial role as partners and providers of care in public health due to their unique ability to tap into faith-based networks and reach marginalized communities.[33]

These organizations can provide significant funding and bring critical awareness for global health activities through their extensive sources of support and donations from religious communities across the world. Although many public health institutions have expressed doubts about collaborating with religious NGOs due to their religious affiliation and the possibility that they might not endorse or implement certain interventions (such as condom use for HIV/AIDS prevention), the invaluable component of sustainability that many religious NGOs bring to the table cannot be denied. Specifically, these religious organizations existed in the community long before any of these epidemics began, and many organizations will remain in the community long after. Faith-based NGOs are most often on the front lines of service, providing much-needed health services, often exceeding the ability of the local government or other governmental organizations.[36]

ACT UP

In the United States, NGOs were also instrumental in the AIDS crisis, particularly with advocacy. ACT UP, or the AIDS Coalition to Unleash Power, is one example of an NGO in the United States that used the power of social pressure to raise awareness about a global health issue and speak out against health injustices.[2] The AIDS crisis produced an upsurge in the amount of global health research, advocacy, and programs. It also increased access for ordinary people to participate in major global health issues and decisions.

In 1987, the FDA granted approval to one of the first AIDS drugs on the market. Costing around $8,000 per year (equivalent to $22,000 in 2024), it was the most expensive drug in history. Activists came together to form ACT UP and protested against the manufacturer, Burroughs Wellcome, on Wall Street. For most people who were HIV positive, this drug was a matter of life and death, yet the price made it inaccessible for most Americans. ACT UP was a nonpartisan group aimed at using direct action to end the AIDS crisis. Through this activism, they were successful in lowering the drug price. Their protest at the New York Stock Exchange stopped trading for the first time in history.

AIDS Epidemic: The Doha Declaration

Within the AIDS epidemic, NGOs have used their skills in public advocacy and lobbying and their economic and intellectual resources to influence policymaking and represent the interests of low-income countries in international debates. One prominent example of this is the role of NGOs in the redefinition of the rules of international intellectual property law in the TRIPS Agreement.[37]

The Agreement on Trade-Related Aspects of Intellectual Property Rights is an international legal recognition of intellectual property and trade between the member organizations of the World Trade Organization. NGOs viewed this agreement as particularly controversial because it allowed corporate monopolies over much-needed medicines and technologies to exist in the name of free trade. This created excessively high prices for patented HIV/AIDS drugs, decreasing the availability of AIDS medicines in low-income countries.

NGOs witnessed millions of African citizens dying due to lack of treatment, which caused public outcry against the World Trade Organization. In 1987, the South African government released the Medicines and Related Substances Control Amendment Act to reduce barriers to affordable HIV/AIDS drugs under the TRIPS Agreement. Soon over 30 pharmaceutical companies challenged this act, stating that it was unconstitutional under the TRIPS Agreement. US pharmaceutical companies convinced the United States to withhold preferential treatment toward South Africa. This led to many influential public health NGOs banding together to launch campaigns against the TRIPS Agreement.[38] Some of these organizations included Doctors Without Borders, Oxfam, Cp Technologies, Health Action International, and Third World Network. The pressure from the NGO advocacy groups and their grassroots campaign brought the criticisms of the TRIPS Agreement to public awareness, creating public outrage and, overall, a public relations disaster for the pharmaceutical companies.

In 2001, President Clinton issued an executive order, promoting the "Accelerating Access Initiative," in which some of the largest pharmaceutical companies were urged to cut the price of HIV/AIDS drugs by

80% for low-income countries. Pressure from the NGO groups led the TRIPS Council to hold a special meeting to reinterpret the TRIPS Agreement, ushering in the creation of the Declaration on the TRIPS Agreement and Public Health.[39] Otherwise known as the Doha Declaration, this clarification of the agreement specifically acknowledges "the gravity of the public health problems afflicting many developing and least-developed countries, especially those resulting from HIV/AIDS, TB, malaria, and other epidemics."[40] In general, this agreement made desperately needed AIDS treatments in lower-income countries more accessible. The campaigns instituted by NGOs garnered much-needed support and global attention to the AIDS crisis. This, in turn, generated international commitments toward strengthening public health support in Africa. Due to NGOs' powerful influence on public opinion, they were able to change policy and the actions of Western states. The Doha Declaration represents the power that NGOs can bring when they come together to represent and fight for public health interests.

From CARE to CARE International

The growth of NGOs has become one of the most influential developments of the 21st century.[21] NGOs have had a unique and increasingly expansive role in global health history, promoting programs to strengthen health systems, long-term collaborative measures, and sustainable practices. NGOs can bring both public and private sector resources together to increase the longevity of programs and be creative with scarce resources. CARE International, which started in World War II, as mentioned earlier, soon grew to be one of the largest NGOs in the world. NGOs like CARE have evolved over time to meet the needs of their beneficiaries and changed their programs to make up for lessons learned. The CARE packages, CARE's main form of aid when it started, were by no means a long-term solution.[10]

In 1955, the food package program was only a small part of the organization's efforts.[1] CARE had expanded to provide general relief to anyone experiencing natural or manmade disasters. At first, CARE's mission was to alleviate hunger, but it quickly learned that the best way to prevent hunger was to construct village water systems, agricultural roads, and overall work on longer-term solutions to poverty. For example, the CARE Plow became popularized in India, when representatives from India told CARE that a plow would dramatically help with their farmers' agriculture production. CARE had researchers, the UN, and Indian agriculturalists design a plow that could be made by local farmers. Even after all these years, they are still made and used in India, where they are known as "CARE plows."

Since CARE was an established organization in international development, other organizations came to it for collaborative efforts and to set up their own aid efforts. MEDICO (Medical International Cooperation Organization), a medical aid program started in the 1950s, was one of CARE's first attempts at improving health among its beneficiaries; it soon became an aspect of every one of CARE's programs. Although MEDICO dissolved in the 1980s, CARE continued to include health programs as one of its primary development activities.

In 1961, when President Kennedy created the Peace Corps, he requested that CARE train the first cohort of volunteers due to its extensive experience in development assistance. CARE started its efforts in community development in Colombia, using that program as a platform as the Peace Corps expanded into other parts of the world. CARE and the Peace Corps would continue to work hand in hand throughout the years.

CARE quickly grew into CARE International when donors in Germany wanted to repay the NGO for the aid it had received in World War II. So German donors raised over $5 million as a thank-you. Recognizing the fundraising potential of international donors, the NGO decided to create CARE Deutschland as the first international member; soon after, more followed. By the end of the 1980s, CARE International had member organizations in Europe, North America, and the Pacific.

In 1993, CARE committed its focus on women and girls as key agents to fight poverty.[41] CARE realized that to address the underlying causes of poverty, it had to strengthen gender equality and women's voice. CARE committed to constantly evaluate its programs and their effectiveness through impact assessments. In 2004, these found that CARE did not give enough attention to women's and girls' rights; five years later, the board decided to put women's and girls' empowerment at the top of its agenda. In 2011, CARE started to incorporate mandatory gender analysis as a design feature in its programs. This is still an uncommon feature for an organization.[42]

Around this time, Dr. Helene Gayle became CEO of CARE and helped to strengthen its long-term impact on sustainable development.[43] Gayle added advocacy as part of CARE's efforts to make more of a difference through policy decisions. She realized that CARE, as one of the world's largest NGOs, held the potential to be a powerful changemaker in global policy. She aimed for the organization to help make the biggest difference in as many people's lives as possible.

CARE was unique because it provided relatively high salaries to its employees compared to other NGOs at the time. This decision helped to reduce turnover rates and increase professionalism and staff expertise. Another unique feature of CARE is that most of its workers are local citizens. For instance, CARE India has trained Indians to run and work the programs; thus, only a few Americans are staffed in this large, countrywide program. In 2016, CARE became one of the first international NGOs to develop monitoring and evaluation tools aligned with the UN's Sustainable Development Goals; these tools helped track an NGO's progress and global influence. CARE identified innovative solutions to provide long-lasting sustainable development, such as creating Village Loans and Savings Associations, or VSLAs. These savings groups brought financial services to rural, low-income areas so that persons with limited access to financial means, such as women, could obtain small loans and increase their ability to make money through entrepreneurial efforts.

CARE has correctly recognized that poverty and health are linked, and that comprehensive capacity-building approaches can effectively improve health outcomes. It views women and girls as the key to overcoming poverty. CARE believes that when women are healthier, their children and families are healthier. It has grown from an emergency relief service to an organization aimed at developing long-lasting solutions to poverty. For instance, it was one of the first programs to develop community-based health projects to stop the incidence of female genital cutting by targeting the social and cultural agents underlying the practice. Previous government or nongovernmental programs had only focused on targeting the health impacts caused by the practice. CARE learned that the community itself must decide to change practices such as this, and that only by creating grassroots advocacy efforts and spaces for public dialogue could this change occur. As in this example, CARE aims to facilitate social change by letting communities lead, rather than by forcing change through its programs. Because of its many years of practicing humanitarian aid, CARE has sharpened its approach, created a niche within the development sector, and specialized its strategies so that other NGOs can follow in its footsteps.

Partners In Health

While CARE International grew to be one of the largest and oldest nonsectarian nongovernmental humanitarian aid organizations, a small NGO on the fringes of Haiti, called Partners In Health (PIH), slowly caught the attention of the world, as it inched its way through one village at a time to eradicate poverty and disease. This organization grew out of a small, one-room clinic in Cange, Haiti's Central Plateau, in 1983 and soon became one of the world's most influential humanitarian organizations.

It all started with Paul Farmer, a soon-to-be medical student at the time of the clinic's founding. While still an undergraduate student at Duke University, Farmer became enthralled with Haitian culture, history, and health when he encountered Haitian migrants at nearby farms. He visited Haiti after graduation and soon found his calling in Cange, where he was astonished by the lack of services and healthcare structure that the community so desperately needed. He then developed a community health program and small clinic.

Cange served as the birthplace of PIH, a home for displaced farmers who had lost their homes when the construction of a nearby dam flooded their valley. There, among some of the poorest and sickest, Farmer found that traditional models of healthcare delivery and finance would not suffice. He and his partners learned how to think outside the box, using both horizontal and vertical measures to deliver services. This was unique: most programs either used horizontal health systems that strengthened measures or vertical strategies, such as programs aimed at a specific disease.

Farmer saw that clinics were ill-equipped to handle the amount of required care and that health centers that *did* have adequate resources were inaccessible to the poor in the countryside. As mentioned in chapter 3 on colonialism, Haiti had suffered colonization, natural disaster, and conflict for most of its history. After colonization, Haiti endured state-sponsored terrorism, supported by the United States. This, as well as US products flooding Haiti's markets, led to hunger, conflict, and political instability. The year 1990 marked the first free elections in Haiti, but by then the country had suffered centuries of misrule and exploitation. As a result of this long history of suffering, it was the poorest country in the Western Hemisphere, according to WHO. In addition to poor health, Haiti lacked adequate sanitation, housing, and basic health infrastructure. As for healthcare workers, most doctors in Haiti had fled after the war for independence. Thus, Farmer's community health development program had to deal with many barriers to work in health equity.

Farmer founded *Zanmi Lasante*, as Partners In Health is known in Haitian Creole, in 1983 along with medical volunteer Ophelia Dahl. In 1987, together with Jim Kim, Farmer's friend (also a physician and anthropologist), Ophelia Dahl, Thomas J. White, and Todd McCormack, PIH was formed in Boston.[2] Farmer traveled back and forth from Harvard in Cambridge to the clinic in Cange, earning his medical degree and PhD in anthropology while helping Zanmi Lasante to grow. He graduated in 1990 from Harvard with some of the top grades in his class, despite having spent most of his time in school volunteering in Cange.

Zanmi Lasante had many lessons to learn as it slowly grew. For example, tuberculosis was one of the leading causes of hospitalization and death in Haiti, but many clinics struggled with treatment failure and drug resistance due to the high number of patients who abandoned treatment.[5] Zanmi Lasante realized that it needed to restructure its programs to deal with TB patients, who lacked necessities such as food or housing. Thus began this NGO's first attempt at a community-based program used to treat a specific disease.

Although the clinics waived fees for patients diagnosed with tuberculosis, many patients had difficulty following up with their care, and many were left partially treated. Zanmi Lasante launched a new strategy that employed the help of *accompagnateurs*, paid community healthcare workers, to provide close support and follow-up for those diagnosed. At first, donors doubted the accompagnateur strategy, as many, such as governmental agencies, hesitated to pay community health workers. Furthermore, earlier work, before Zanmi Lasante, attributed Haiti's low adherence to treatment to cultural explanations such as sorcery or inability to tell time. Zanmi Lasante tested its new program by providing the standard form of care to certain sectors, while employing the new accompagnateur strategy to others. Those diagnosed with tuberculosis were enrolled in a program involving daily visits from their local health worker, financial assistance, and nutritional supplements. The program was so successful that the accompagnateur strategy became a standard part of the NGO's care: it was integrated into other programs, such as its AIDS treatment programs. Community workers made sure that patients took their medicines, had access to food, and were not subject to barriers such as transportation costs that blocked their access to care.

PIH in Boston helped raise money to fund not only Zanmi Lasante in Haiti but also other programs in the world. Zanmi Lasante soon expanded to become the largest healthcare provider in Haiti outside of the government. Its success in Haiti inspired other countries, such as Rwanda, Peru, and Russia, to request PIH to establish services and programs there as well.

When the government of Rwanda invited this NGO to expand its services to that country in 2005, PIH proved that comprehensive healthcare could be delivered even in the poorest of districts. Rwanda lay in ruins from war and had one of the highest rates of child mortality globally when PIH workers arrived. Workers from Haiti came to train local healthcare workers and recruit staff. Other NGOs in Rwanda were mostly concentrated in cities; rural areas were left without any system of healthcare. PIH implemented its standard of accompagnateur care, looking to local knowledge and inequitable barriers to healthcare to inform the creation of its programs. By paying and training local community health workers, it could create jobs for the poor while also increasing the effectiveness of medical treatments, such as increasing adherence to antiretroviral therapy. Paying healthcare workers proved to be cheaper than providing second-line HIV/AIDS medications. PIH created a sustainable system of care by working closely with local doctors, the ministry of health, and the government of Rwanda. Soon, the entire program was run by the ministry of health in Rwanda; its mission was to address more long-term health issues of its citizens.

PIH works to target structural barriers to healthcare while training locals to work closely with their neighbors, ensuring that they had the needed tools to conquer disease and poverty.[44] The concept of accompagnateurs and accompaniment made the NGO famous, with its model of healthcare service delivery and its aim to work closely with the public sector. PIH recognized that only the government had the ability to make long-term commitments to its citizens and the healthcare system. By strengthening existing healthcare structures, providing close support for the ill, and involving the community at every stage of design and evaluation of programs, this NGO has identified a method that can comprehensively deliver healthcare while providing long-term solutions for the poor. While earlier policymakers and public health officials had discredited the idea that antiretroviral therapy could be provided in low-income setting such as Rwanda, due to the non-Western means of "telling time," PIH proved that a system of full support, daily visits, and close monitoring by local health workers could lead to higher levels of patients staying with their course of treatment.

The main lesson that NGOs such as PIH teach us is that we must meet patients where they are instead of expecting them to come to the ones providing the service. Farmer explained that

> to accompany someone is to go somewhere with him or her, to break bread together, to be present on a journey with a beginning and an end. There's an element of mystery, of openness, of trust, in accompaniment. The companion, the *accompagnateur*, says "I'll go with you and support you on your journey wherever it leads."[45]

This type of thinking moves away from short-term, Band-Aid solutions to long-lasting relationships with the community.

PIH believes that the true measure of success for a health program is a renewed faith in the healthcare system itself.[46] While other programs may have used community health workers to complement their care, this NGO emphasized a new concept of training workers for long-term service and embracing them as professional members of the healthcare service delivery. Some other NGOs refused to directly work with the governments in their host country, due to claims of corruption; however, PIH challenged this notion, stating that any organization truly interested in creating lasting change will work directly with the government, involve officials at every stage, and train local citizens to become a part of the work. A hospital director working after the earthquake in Haiti in 2010 claimed that "it was an unusual experience, the help from Zanmi Lasante. I had them join my managerial team and discuss how to handle a difficult situation. It is the first time I had this kind of relationship with an NGO."[47] PIH shows us that by providing proper care to those in need, from hospitals all the way into patients' homes, we can eradicate poverty one paid community health worker at a time.

The Bangladesh Rural Advancement Committee

Unlike the previous NGOs founded by Westerners, the Bangladesh Rural Advancement Committee (BRAC) was founded and run by

Bangladeshis. Born in the aftermath of the Liberation War, BRAC was a small, temporary relief operation that soon grew to be one of the largest NGOs in the world.

It all started in 1970, when Fazle Hasan Abed, a businessman working for Shell Oil, opened his house for survivors of Tropical Cyclone Nora, one of the worst storms in history. Soon after the cyclone, Bangladesh (East Pakistan at the time) found itself entrenched in a revolution, soon declaring itself separate from Pakistan. Abed fled to England and quit his position at Shell, denouncing the Pakistani chairman for using him in the war.[48] Jobless and demonstrating in front of embassies, Abed rallied others to help him raise funds for his war-torn country. He returned with funds to Bangladesh to form BRAC, then known as the Bangladesh Rehabilitation Assistance Committee. Even though his organization had no track record and fewer than 10 employees, he convinced Oxfam to fund his first proposal for rehabilitation projects. BRAC was so successful that it had over £15,000 left over after the project and offered to pay Oxfam back. Oxfam—perplexed, as it had never encountered such a situation—told the new NGO to put the money toward its next program. BRAC realized that its operation would be more than a temporary assistance program, so, in 1974, Abed changed the name to Bangladesh Rural Advancement Committee.

In BRAC's first proposal, Abed wrote that "the struggle for liberation brought about a new climate, a new awareness, and a desire for change." At the time, Bangladesh was the poorest country on earth. Eighty percent of the population was illiterate. So, some of BRAC's first programs were educational because it recognized that education was a foundation for development.

BRAC started research to learn about its poorest citizens and found that some of the poorest were women, obscured by purdah, a type of formal segregation that kept them confined inside their homes. BRAC's early research uncovered a harsh side of life in Bangladesh: it was the only country in the world in which men outlived women. From its inception, BRAC realized that to make a difference, it had to target poor women and create gender-sensitive programs. It started to almost exclusively recruit women under 30 from the project areas and trained them extensively. In fact, BRAC was almost unique among NGOs because it was not afraid to fire incompetent staff and hire new employees. At the time, this strategy was seen as harsh. BRAC also put a major focus on constantly retraining, creating jobs, hiring women, and avoiding the phenomenon of "parachuting in" employees from the West. Because it solely recruited local staff, it benefited from developing a mutual trust and faith that success is possible.

One of the defining programs of BRAC is its microfinance program. At the time of its founding, Abed was able to build on the experience of Ela Bhatt, who had started a bank with microfinancing for the Self Employed Women's Association (SEWA) in Gujarat, India, in 1974 (Bill Foege, pers. comm., 2023). BRAC's early research found that villagers took out loans only for trading purposes and that entrepreneurial activities barely existed. BRAC realized that if the poor could be connected to the mainstream economy through employment and skills building, they could eliminate poverty. Thus, the NGO started creating Village Organizations, in which villagers of similar backgrounds could be trained in various skills and choose to participate in income-generating activities. BRAC offers two types of loans for the poor. The first is a small loan given only to women for small agricultural, livestock, or handicraft operations. The second is a larger loan, given to either men or women who were denied loans from the traditional finance system to fund small enterprises.

While most microenterprise programs gave the poor the financial means to create income-generating activities, these programs did not provide them with the educational means, which often drove the poor into petty commerce or household production. BRAC prides itself on its extensive training and market research to find economic opportunities. For instance, in 1983, it consulted women on their existing income-generating activities and found that poultry rearing was popular, but high poultry mortality was common. BRAC then trained a village volunteer to vaccinate the poultry, giving the volunteer a small loan to buy the vaccines and get her started. This approach created employment opportunities for villagers while helping women make more money in the activities in which they were already engaged.

Although microfinance has been conventionally targeted at adults, BRAC recognized the growing number of adolescents in South Asia and decided to use this population as a catalyst for social change and economic growth. Most development efforts either focused on children or adults, so BRAC decided to create an economic empowerment program for adolescent girls that would offer skills trainings, savings groups, and access to small loans. Furthermore, BRAC opened up its own university, dedicated to educating the next generation's leaders and encouraging them to engage in careers in national development.[49]

BRAC found that some of the main reasons for poverty and defaults on loans were ill health and sickness. Through BRAC's microfinance program, it trained village members in essential healthcare, so they could volunteer their services by providing basic health information and services in their allocated areas.[50] The volunteers could make money by selling medicines and referring the sick to clinics. BRAC soon expanded its health programs and included basic health information and training as part of its credit programs. The NGO found that this credit program–based, health-education approach was far more effective than other campaigns because it targeted the poor, women, and others who traditionally were not exposed to most educational or media campaigns. The main strategy used by BRAC was to employ health workers and to increase community participation, which led to increased "ownership" of the programs and, thus, sustainability.[51] BRAC's Oral Therapy Extension Program, aimed at eliminating waterborne illnesses, treated over 12 million households from 1981 to 1990 alone.[48]

BRAC has used a heavily integrated monitoring and evaluation system in all of its activities to learn from mistakes and improve effectiveness. Since its inception, this NGO has been brutally honest in reports—citing its failures—and has been committed to listening to its citizens.[52] In 1975, BRAC created a separate division for research and learning, which has now grown into the country's largest research institution.[53] Its research found that its programs, as with those of most NGOs, did not reach the ultra-poor, the poorest section of the population with few or no asset base.[54] Although microfinance targeted the poor, the ultra-poor were reluctant to borrow and more likely to drop out of such programs if they did join. BRAC decided to create programs specifically designed to reach this segment of the population through promotional schemes such as asset grants and protective measures (e.g., stipends and healthcare services). As food insecurity was one of the main causes of poverty, BRAC collaborated with the World Food Programme to provide food rations in addition to the microfinance programs so that the ultra-poor would participate and also save some income, without fear of losing their few assets.[52]

Unlike other NGOs, BRAC has succeeded in creating social enterprises so that 76% of its budget is self-financed and sustainable.[49] Indeed, the organization was awarded the highest credit rating by the Credit Rating Agency of Bangladesh Ltd. It has learned to use innovative practices and production-lowering techniques to lower its costs and risk of dependency on aid or grants. BRAC was quoted by the *Economist* as being "the largest, fastest-growing non-governmental organisation (NGO) in the world—and one of the most businesslike."[55] Now BRAC operates in nine countries in Asia and Africa, which allows the organization to use its extensive development experience in other low-income settings. This NGO promoted South-to-South assistance and was a pioneer in developing indigenous public health programs.

Orbis International

While NGOs like CARE or BRAC use comprehensive strategies to solve multiple public health issues, other NGOs focus on one single issue and specialize in one type of strategy. One of the key strengths of NGOs is that they are adaptive and innovative. Orbis International is a key example of innovation and resiliency, using the tools it has on hand to give care in the field. It is skilled at using few resources or building on local resources to create its interventions. NGOs often use new strategies to deliver health services and can be creative in situations where other agencies cannot.

Orbis International is a global health nonprofit that has creatively used its resources to deliver health services around the world. Unlike

CARE International and other similar NGOs that deliver a wide range of services to strengthen health systems, this NGO focuses specifically on targeting and specializing in a specific public health issue. Orbis is dedicated to fighting blindness by bringing together partners and medical professionals to treat patients and train healthcare workers. It has converted an aircraft into a training center and clinic, with the passenger cabin transformed into a teaching room and another cabin for an eye exam room.[7] The plane is stocked with teaching materials, medical equipment, and more than 150 tapes on eye treatment. When Orbis is invited by a country's local ophthalmology society, a team of doctors, nurses, technicians, and staff arrive, bringing medical equipment with them. They focus on training and mentoring local doctors and healthcare workers to treat eye diseases. Since 1982, this NGO has provided treatment and training in over 92 countries.

Modern-Day Partnerships in Global Health

UNHCR and NGOs

In some global health crises, operations would be unsuccessful without NGOs. They can be seen as the building blocks within a particular intervention. The partnership with UNHCR is one of those instances. The UNHCR that we see today operates completely differently from the one that was established 70 years ago. Refugee protection was originally considered the responsibility of lawyers. UNHCR was established so that it could advocate international refugee law and provide legal assistance.[56] It was not created to engage in humanitarian aid or provide global health assistance.

When Europeans no longer required assistance after World War II, UNHCR turned to other refugee crises, such as those in the continent of Africa. It realized that these new types of refugees in low-income countries did not require *legal* assistance, but *material* assistance. The conventional screening of refugees by legal status was then adapted with the help of NGOs to determine the health needs of refugees instead. NGOs including Oxfam, Doctors Without Borders, and Save the

Children helped to develop tools to triage, or sort, populations according to need. NGOs, particularly medical ones, helped to shift UNHCR's focus to the health needs of the population. Thus, unlike the original approach for UNHCR to target refugees, this approach emphasized the mission to target *humans* instead. Now, UNHCR classifies refugees according to their needs, such as "unaccompanied children," "single heads of household," "survivors of rape," and so on.[57] The influence of NGOs to adopt the new classification system and emphasis on health needs has transformed UNHCR into an organization known for responding to the most dire refugee crises in the world.

UNHCR and NGOs cannot operate without each other. Their collaboration is one of the most unique partnerships among the UN agencies—indeed, among most agencies in the world. They have created a formal partnership that allows both actors to perform their functions as equal partners.[18] Through years of informal collaboration with UNHCR, NGOs advocated to create a formal partnership called the Partnership in Action Conference, which led to the Declaration and a Plan of Action in 1994. This partnership lays out a set of guidelines and a framework for cooperation so that NGOs can help create funding proposals and implement programs, instead of acting as subcontractors. The traditional structure that placed NGOs in a subordinate position under UN agencies was turned on its head with this new partnership agreement. UNHCR now acts as a strong agency that coordinates the efforts of NGOs to avoid repetition or competition between programs. It also coordinates the presence of NGOs and the government, so that NGOs can implement their programs without any interference. It acts as an intermediary between the government, the international donor community, and the NGO community so that it can translate missions and funds into on-the-ground action.

NGOs are key to operations within refugee camps, often filling in the gaps where UNHCR cannot operate and advocating for the needs of the refugees.[58] UNHCR recognizes NGOs' invaluable role, even awarding the high honor of the Nansen Refugee Award to Doctors Without Borders in 1993.[18] NGOs are everywhere where UNHCR is present, helping to turn every UNHCR plan of action into reality.

NGOs are the first ones to react and spot human rights injustices or health emergencies, which they report to UNHCR. And since this organization cannot be everywhere at once, it relies on NGOs to provide this feedback as well as their local expertise to relate to the refugees in need. NGOs also can work in dangerous and hard-to-reach areas and are often the first ones to receive the refugees and respond in crises. Without the traditional bureaucratic structure, they can act quickly as well as lobby for the fair treatment of refugees in conflicts. These NGOs cannot act alone, however, because most of their funding is from UNHCR. This, in turn, keeps NGOs accountable through strict reporting structures for the disbursement of funds.

DADAAB REFUGEE CAMP

One example of the contribution of NGOs to refugee health and well-being is the Dadaab refugee complex, in Kenya. This camp houses generations of refugees and was once the largest refugee camp in the world.[59] Its growth largely stems from the government's strict policies against refugee settlement in the country. Although NGOs did not possess the ability to help settle the refugees into their host country, they were able to stop the closure of the camp, which would have forced nearly 100,000 refugees back to Somalia, where they would be killed in the civil war or droughts. NGO aid was crucial in assisting these refugees for over two decades, helping to sustain the camp as it grew. NGOs helped to establish clinics, schools, and food distribution centers in partnership with trained refugee community workers.

In 2016, the Kenyan government threatened to close the camp because of terrorism attacks linked to al-Qaeda and the Islamic State, and the unfair accusation that the Somali refugees had perpetrated them. Immediately after this announcement, NGOs such as Amnesty International, Doctors Without Borders, and World Vision Kenya lobbied against the government's decision.[60,61] UNHCR and the government of Kenya were working to repatriate the refugees; however, NGOs investigated and found that this "voluntary repatriation" was not voluntary at all: the refugees were, in fact, fearful of violence and lack of food and healthcare if they returned home.

The NGOs committed themselves to helping the government provide a sustainable plan of action to integrate the refugees into Kenyan society.[59] These actions prompted the High Court of Kenya to rule, in 2017, that its decision to close the camp was unconstitutional and discriminatory toward refugees. Since then, Kenya has adopted the Comprehensive Refugee Response Framework, which was proposed by the United Nations.[62] This framework provided a plan for governments, stakeholders, and organizations to provide host countries with the support they needed to aid refugees as well as to integrate them into society. Although this plan is still being implemented, Dadaab refugee camp has provided other refugee camps with cutting-edge solutions toward health, humanitarianism, and sustainability. For example, although the Kenyan government and UNHCR are in charge of the camp, it is mostly run by democratically elected camp volunteers, working hand in hand with NGOs. Dadaab was one of the first camps in the world to operate this way.

This type of sustainable leadership, as well as the strong infrastructure that the aid organizations have provided, has led others to rethink the way other refugee camps around the world should be established. While NGOs such as CARE International or PIH provide long-term structural programs to address the roots of poverty, other NGOs are adept at providing emergency assistance or immediate problem-solving to fill in the gaps of governments or other government agencies.

NGOs in Pandemic Response

In times of crisis, governments tend to have systems in place to respond to public needs. However, transitioning of resources, commitments toward improving health quality, and reduced budgets in the 1990s resulted in governments reaching out to international NGOs for help. Alma-Ata, a joint declaration under the auspices of WHO in 1978, recognized the importance of primary healthcare for all populations globally.[29] In it, several articles mention the participation of the public in areas of health, such as increasing community participation and empowering individuals in public health. The increasing number of health concerns, particularly emergencies, epidemics, and pandemics, has created a strain on national governments, which made the intervention of NGO emergency and pandemic response attractive.

NGOs tend to understand the local context and norms of a particular culture and region, an integral step to developing a comprehensive pandemic response.[63] Local NGOs have close relationships with the community, and international NGOs have resources and technical assistance that can bolster local responses. With regard to existing government responses, NGOs play a critical role in implementing structured health programs and responses. In nonemergency settings, NGOs strengthen existing healthcare structures to improve access to and quality of care, providing a foundation during pandemics. In emergency settings, NGOs act on the front line by establishing medical facilities, providing supplies to victims, and supporting local public health responses. One type of NGO response reflects disaster management and relief. Some are traditional relief agencies, and others act as public service contractors on behalf of international organizations. Another type of NGO is one that uses community-based approaches to mitigate disasters and prepare for emergencies.

During the Ebola outbreak in Sierra Leone in 2014, NGOs helped to support the government while also coordinating local response capacity.[64] NGOs increased the number of beds in health facilities and built Ebola treatment centers. International NGOs, such as Doctors Without Borders, helped to provide primary healthcare by contributing medical professionals and other health infrastructures. NGOs engaged in activities such as health education, training of local health staff, and providing sanitation and water—which all helped to leverage other public health responses. The Ebola crisis highlighted the importance of creating a multisector response, especially with respect to the high threat to national security.

During the COVID-19 pandemic, governments were essential in fighting the pandemic; however, NGOs were also instrumental in providing needed services.[65] Although COVID-19 has biological origins, it is also a social problem with social consequences. COVID-19 is exacerbated by social factors such as food culture, lifestyle, and social communication. Lack of knowledge on the ways in which the virus is transmitted contributes to its spread. NGOs help to increase public awareness, provide services for vulnerable groups, and advocate changes in social policies. NGOs are useful when working in community-based surveillance, providing disease control tools with community partners, and facilitating collaboration between public health officials and staff on the ground.[66] Some NGOs have worked with media outlets to prevent the spread of misinformation about the virus. Others adapted their existing programs to ensure that much-needed services were maintained during the pandemic. Some NGOs worked to mitigate secondary impacts of the pandemic, such as gender-based violence, the spread of communicable diseases, or loss of maternal health services for pregnant women afraid to access health services. Other NGOs have worked to reach remote communities through existing relationships with local leaders.

Countries have struggled to manage the COVID-19 outbreak alone; however, successful countries have used the abilities of other sectors. A multisectoral approach to pandemic preparedness and response is critical, and NGOs often play an important role in bridging the gap between knowledge and practice in the field. As COVID-19 continues to play a role in major public health responses today, we must recognize the contributions of all sectors and their strengths and weaknesses.

The Role of NGOs in Global Health Today

The NGOs presented in this chapter are only a few out of thousands in our current global health landscape. These NGOs represent a diverse number of global health interventions, priorities, and interests. Each provides a different function within the vast network of public health aid. Now more than ever, we need innovative strategies, quick organizational responses, and community-based grassroots interventions within the field of global health. The rise of NGOs in recent years has created both advantages and challenges for global health.

The large number of NGOs has led to competition for funding and sometimes redundancies in programmatic efforts. However, as NGOs become global, they are held to higher standards of quality and effectiveness. Now, NGOs are held accountable by beneficiaries and donors through evaluation, internal and external audits, and assessment processes. In 1997, for instance, a global network called the Structural Adjustment Participatory Review Initiative (SAPRI) was established to promote and evaluate economic reform.[21] Other programs, such as NGO Watch, have been launched to provide reviews, critiques, and evaluations of NGOs and their programs.[8] In 2004, five US NGOs, including Save the Children and World Vision, decided to have their programs evaluated by two independent auditing agencies.[13] More NGOs were quick to follow. NGO transparency is gained through these standards of effectiveness as well as through the sheer mass of public support. NGOs have also been subject to more and more research with the rise of randomized clinical trials and other studies that have been popularized through public health research.[67]

It would be remiss to ignore the faults of NGOs within global health history. The main problem for NGOs is that they are dependent on donors for funding, which may dictate their missions or timelines. This dependence on donors leads some organizations to become large fundraising institutions, with most of their efforts spent on raising money or applying for grants.

NGOs may undermine local development or may have unequal power relations with local leaders.[68] One example of such a failure was in Haiti after the 2010 earthquake. NGOs came to the aid of citizens, providing shelters and support; however, the aid they pledged to the country soon dried up, leading to only short-term programs. This Band-Aid approach led many to remain in extreme poverty and homeless. Many NGOs were criticized for not hiring locals and hiring highly paid non-Haitian staff members. Others wondered whether the presence of so many NGOs held the country back from developing its own infrastructure and economy by flooding the market with emergency relief funds.

NGOs may support existing hierarchies and may decrease opportunities for local participation. Some communities may not even have direct contact with NGO directors, and NGOs may have top-heavy leadership structures. Thus, NGOs must be structured to disrupt imperialist strategies, employ locals, and have equal footing with local leadership.

Although NGOs have many weaknesses, like any other approach to global health, one of their main strengths is how adaptive and dynamic they can be. NGOs have become popular in many global health contexts because of their ability to adapt to any setting, try new methods, and listen to the public. As people's trust in the government has declined, more faith has been placed in the hands of NGOs to solve our world's most pressing health crises. Not only have NGOs been popularized with the public through advocacy, fundraising, and raising awareness, but they have also been progressively favored over governmental agencies by donors due to the increasing recognition of the government's failures in aid and development. In many public health responses, NGOs are seen as the neutral voice that the community trusts. Governments are increasingly outsourcing their programs to NGOs, particularly noncore functions. In other areas, some countries prefer to channel development aid through NGOs rather than through local governments in which the fear of misuse of assistance is high.[5] While some NGOs' missions are directly supported by the government, others are created because they do not think the government is doing enough in an area, while even others act in direct opposition of the government (e.g., Planned Parenthood).[14] Through the wide diversity of NGOs and their unique ability to mobilize communities, NGOs have become a key part in the aid chain of global health.[4]

They have become increasingly professional and specialized, now requiring their staff to have higher levels of education and their programs to have higher levels of compliance. NGOs act as intermediaries between governments and communities, often promoting local involvement and acting in nonpartisan measures without any political affiliations. NGOs are adept at bringing public and private partners together while collaborating across multiple sectors. No matter where a global health crisis occurs, NGOs are present. With their local knowledge and ability to reach vulnerable populations, NGOs are at the heart of every major intervention.

Concluding Thoughts

BILL FOEGE

These NGOs represent a diverse number of global health interventions, priorities, and interests. Each NGO provides a different function within the vast network of public health aid. The rapid development of NGOs has improved global health significantly. In general, this has had a major and positive impact on global health equity and the ability to reach the poorest in each society. NGOs may be second only to political involvement in their potential to improve global health.

Are there drawbacks to NGOs? Small organizations often lack economies of scale. At times, as in disaster situations, the number of groups responding can make an organized response difficult for the country with the disaster. On the other hand, NGOs allow many more people to become involved in global health problems. The coordination of so many diverse groups may be a problem, but the positives certainly outweigh the negatives.

CHAPTER 10

Hybrid Organizations

BILL FOEGE

W e've discussed global, bilateral, multilateral, and NGO (nongov-ernmental) programs. The latest major participants in global health are hybrid programs. These overlap multilateral and NGO pro-grams but are becoming more powerful and more effective in deliver-ing global health improvements.

Forty years ago, it was apparent that competition between programs could be harmful, even when the participants were absolutely com-mitted to the same outcomes. It has been mentioned, for example, that some programs were jealous of the involvement of the World Bank in health programs. The Bank had such prestige and power that coun-tries could be more responsive to Bank ideas than those from the World Health Organization (WHO).

The most significant chasm developed as WHO, headed by Half-dan Mahler, promoted the improvement of health systems, while UNICEF, headed by Jim Grant, was promoting specific interventions. Both agency leaders were people of great compassion and drive, fo-cused on improving global health. However, they appeared to have little interest in coordinating their approaches.

A breakthrough occurred when Jonas Salk began talking with Ken Warren at the Rockefeller Foundation. Immunization was one of the four priorities at UNICEF at the time, and WHO had invested in the Expanded Program on Immunization, attempting to provide the basic childhood immunizations as a follow-up to the successful smallpox-eradication program. Could this be used as a way to form a coalition?

With the support of Robert McNamara, former president of the World Bank, the Rockefeller Foundation agreed to assemble the key immunization programs in the world for a discussion at its Bellagio, Italy, facility. Interest was high, and soon the heads of UNICEF, WHO, the World Bank, United Nations Development Programme (UNDP), and USAID—plus researchers, academics, and experienced immunization leaders—had agreed to attend.

Before the meeting, Jim Grant and Halfdan Mahler became invested in the idea and came to talk to me. Their question was whether I would agree to head up a task force if the meeting reached the conclusion that one would be useful. They emphasized that they both had strong egos but were willing to take a chance if I would lead the task force. They had two caveats. One, I would never use the word *coordinate* as it would be a nonstarter for each organization. They did not want to be coordinated. We agreed on the word *facilitate*. The second admonishment was that I would be willing to assume a low profile if things worked—and perhaps a larger profile if they didn't work!

The Bellagio participants presented much pushback to the idea of a task force. The argument was that one more organization could only reduce the efficiency of the effort. But Grant and Mahler were now united, and the meeting ended with agreement for a task force to facilitate immunization.

This is not the place to review the incredible cooperation that developed with quarterly meetings of WHO, UNICEF, UNDP, the World Bank, and the Rockefeller Foundation. The meetings reviewed progress, identified obstacles to improvement, and delegated responsibility to seek corrections. Periodically, a global meeting of a hundred or more would report on progress and seek input on other ideas. Such meetings were held in Colombia, India, Thailand, and France.

Improvement was so dramatic that, on September 30, 1990, Jim Grant announced at a UN Children's Summit that 80% of the children of the world had received at least one vaccine. (In 1983, the immunization rate had been approximately 20% globally.) Grant called the joint effort to immunize children the greatest peacetime effort ever seen. Clearly, the task force was the most successful hybrid program at the time. Yet no single global agency was in charge: *cooperation came from people agreeing to an outcome rather than a structure.*[1]

A second factor in promoting hybrid programs came with the successful Mectizan program, which started in 1985 with Merck's gift of this drug, for free, to fight river blindness. This effort eventually incorporated the global agencies but, again, answered to none of them. Earlier efforts to have WHO and USAID involved had not been successful. Then Merck offered the Task Force for Child Survival the same condition offered to WHO and USAID: that the company would provide Mectizan free if the agencies would develop a program of distribution. The task force agreed, and as mentioned in chapter 13, decisions were made by a Mectizan Expert Committee, independent of outside influence. (Chapter 13, on pharmaco-philanthropy, also details the continued contributions of the Task Force for Global Health in the last 40 years.)

Success was rapid, and every goal was exceeded. Soon, WHO and others were asking to be part of the program. It is the most unique hybrid program in global health. Merck has now contributed in excess of 5 billion free treatments. Blindness from onchocerciasis has decreased dramatically. Indeed, discussions now center around eradication of the problem, rather than just control.

The past two decades have seen an explosion of effective hybrid programs. One such program, the Global Alliance for Vaccines and Immunization (Gavi) has changed global immunization, combining efforts of global agencies, pharmaceutical companies, foundations, private agencies, and governments.

In addition, there are now programs for lymphatic filariasis (combining the efforts of two pharmaceutical companies), micronutrients, childhood worm reduction, hepatitis control, trachoma, and other often neglected diseases. All involve public and private agencies as well as commercial companies.

It is likely that these programs are mapping the future of global health. We still need WHO, UNICEF, and other global and bilateral agencies, but hybrid organizations are bringing new passion and resources to supplement the traditional agencies.

CHAPTER 11

Early Philanthropy and the Rockefeller Foundation

KIERA CHAN

The COVID-19 pandemic demonstrated the strengths and weaknesses of global health. Once, public health was largely ignored, especially on a global scale. At the beginning of the 20th century, however, it was pushed to the forefront of the international agenda by a single organization, the Rockefeller Foundation.[1]

Emergence of Philanthropy in the United States

The Oxford English Dictionary defines *philanthropy* as the desire to promote the welfare of others; it is often described as the desire to promote the common good.[2] Before the Industrial Revolution, this desire was often expressed as charity, with uncoordinated acts of volunteerism and almsgiving, primarily by religious groups. At the end of the 19th century, charities started to donate in more systematic ways and with a more business-like approach. Business titans such as John D. Rockefeller led this shift.[3] The Industrial Revolution, itself, brought many advances in technology as well as a surge in resources.[4] With the invention of steam power, improved iron production, and the advent of mechanized factories, production of consumer goods increased and prices decreased. This brought not only a higher standard of living for many, but also immense wealth for a few, including Andrew Carnegie and John D. Rockefeller.[5]

The Industrial Revolution also ushered in urbanization and overcrowding, which led to more diseases, orphans, widows, and refugees.[6] Conversely, the revolution also created better modes of communication and transportation, which facilitated the transfer of ideas and distribution of aid.

Philanthropy increased with the advocacy for causes such as the abolitionist, temperance, and women's movements.[7] During this time, the need for social reform accelerated. This, in turn, conflicted with the current political culture, and government was unable to address this need. In particular, federalism of the 19th century caused conflicts among citizens about giving the government the authority to set standards of social well-being across the United States.[6] Within this gap, philanthropy increased; modern foundations, as we know them, were created. Although the Rockefeller Foundation was not the first of its kind, it was the major foundation of the century to revolutionize the field of public health.[8] Rockefeller called this "the business of benevolence" and proposed foundations as the answer for distributing great wealth.[9]

Scientific Giving

Andrew Carnegie was a son of poor, Scottish immigrants, who dominated the steel industry. Eventually, he founded the Carnegie Corporation of New York.[4] He soon became the second richest man in America. At the time of the Industrial Revolution, the American public had become accustomed to the excess riches of the so-called robber barons, who had become wealthy due to corrupt practices in the industry.[10] Thus, when Carnegie wrote his manifesto, "The Gospel of Wealth," the public was astounded. He wrote that the rich should devote themselves to giving and had a responsibility to spend their money to benefit the greater good of society.[9] He proposed a new type of philanthropy, in which the wealthy had to oversee the distribution of their wealth and avoid sporadic forms of charity or what he saw as "handouts" to the poor. This inspired a new type of giving—called "scientific giving"—in which the root causes of poverty were targeted instead of its symptoms.[11] Carnegie saw the latter as perpetuating a state of dependence on aid due to the "idleness" of the poor. His scientific approach to philanthropy became popular, leading to the reform of private and public welfare. Carnegie thought that handouts to the poor, without particular attention to the root causes of poverty, would do more harm than good. He wrote that "he who dies rich, dies disgraced."[4]

Modern Philanthropy

This new type of philanthropy was invested in the ideology of the Progressive Era.[1] This new philosophy embraced the values of Protestantism as well as the rationality of science and social sciences. Protestant values were infused in the social movements of the day because reformers believed that Christians should apply their teachings to social reform. The social changes brought by the Industrial Revolution and large-scale industrial capitalism led to new techniques in education and organization.

Meanwhile, the middle class of this era was becoming increasingly professionalized. This era accepted capitalism but focused its attention on the social problems of the day. These features brought in Rockefeller's new type of philanthropy, which applied scientific strategies and organized solutions. Because the traditional modes of charity could not achieve the aims of the Progressive Era and the wealthy were making more than they could give away, the new generation of philanthropists sought to apply their strategies of business toward giving. This scientific and business-like approach emphasized the role of education, research, and efficiency.[9] Foundations started to award grants, which helped to create links among philanthropists, researchers, government, and public organizations. Trusts were created for specific purposes. They were designed to target a particular issue, such as education or health, and created for specific periods of time to work in that area.[6] Overall, the rise of professionalism and reform allowed philanthropists to reform their ways of giving to align with the modern ideologies of that time.

The Start of the Rockefeller Foundation

In 1913, John D. Rockefeller established the Rockefeller Foundation, which soon became the most well-known philanthropic organization in the world.[8] He became the richest man in the world within a span of only 40 years, leading to his retirement as the head of Standard Oil. His fortune grew even after his retirement, owing to the oil shares he owned and the demand for oil created by the automobile.[9]

Rockefeller, a Baptist, was interested in philanthropy even from an early age.[1] For example, as a teenager he saved money from his first job to donate to the church. However, by the 1890s, the sheer size of his fortune made it impossible to donate through charity. He was badgered and harassed wherever he went: people followed him, pleading for money for what they regarded as good causes.

Fueled by a need for a vision of giving, he found a full-time philanthropic adviser, Frederick T. Gates.[9] Gates was an ordained minister and was serving as the head of the American Baptist Education Society at the time. Rockefeller's son, John D. Rockefeller Jr., and Gates worked to change the face of philanthropy and revamped Rockefeller's previous efforts at personal charity into an organized, institutional operation, which reflected the current corporate business practices of the day. The two men aimed to use scientific giving to tackle areas of need that the government had traditionally neglected, such as education, public health, and agriculture. Gates told Rockefeller Senior that his fortune was increasing at a quick pace and that he must keep up with it or else "it will crush you and your children and your children's children."[11] Gates's approach to philanthropy was on a scale parallel to the oil trust that had made it possible. Gates soon turned Rockefeller's seemingly arbitrary acts of charity into an organized central system for distributing funds to causes that aligned with the foundation's mission. This type of system became the groundwork for all of the subsequent Rockefeller philanthropies.

The Foundation's Entry into Public Health

Modern public health can be dated to 1796, when Dr. Edward Jenner gave the first smallpox vaccination to James Phipps. The US Public Health Service had its origins in the creation of Marine Hospitals two years later, in 1798. In 1799, the Massachusetts Legislature enacted America's first board of health in Boston; Paul Revere was its first president. Many states soon followed this precedent, and the American Public Health Association was formed in 1872 to provide for an interchange of skills and knowledge by all public health workers.

International public health, which would evolve into modern global health, was given a major boost by the first International Sanitary Conference, in 1851.[12] This was followed by 11 more conferences over 50 years and the eventual creation of an agency called the Office International d'Hygiène Publique in Paris, in 1907.[8]

The Rockefeller Foundation was intent on providing leadership and resources to this growing movement. At the same time, philanthropy was seen as a means to counter working-class unrest and to calm threats to business interests. Countering criticism and protecting resources from taxation were also motives, as negative publicity for the Rockefellers was at its height during this time.[12]

As journalists highlighted the monopolies of the company and linked business interests with philanthropic interests, the Rockefeller family was pushed toward finding a neutral ground in which to pursue philanthropy. The neutral area in which it could fund operations that did not directly link to its business interests fell within the realm of international public health. Frederick Gates pushed the Foundation toward medicine after he read William Osler's 1892 text, *The Principles and Practices of Medicine*.[8] Gates was surprised that, although the book detailed diagnostic criteria, no research existed on the causes of conditions. He realized how neglected the study of medicine was at the time, so he decided that establishing an institute solely dedicated to medical research would be his first step as adviser.

The Rockefeller Institute for Medical Research

At this time in the early 1900s, although medical practice dated back several thousand years, there were few standards and scarce research in the United States to understand the causes of diseases and their best treatments. This knowledge gap provided an opportunity for the Rockefeller Foundation to test its insights into scientific giving by investing in education and research. Later named Rockefeller University, the Rockefeller Institute for Medical Research, created in 1901,[8] was the first American organization dedicated to medical research. The death of Rockefeller's grandson from scarlet fever in 1901 was the catalyst for the effort.[13]

During this era, infectious diseases were considered the primary menace to human health. Rockefeller followed the paths of research institutions in Europe, which were applying laboratory science toward research on infectious diseases. One of the institute's first projects was the milk survey, in 1901.[14] In New York City, the rise of industrialization and urbanization increased infection rates, leading to high rates of infant mortality. One of the scientific directors at the board of health saw that this was linked with the city's milk supply and received a grant from the Rockefeller Institute to investigate the association. The grant funded a survey of milk supply and distribution, which revealed that bacteria were being spread in unsanitary facilities. This finding led to the training of farm staff in sterilization methods.

Publication of the survey results led to a public outcry, inspiring the city to create new positions for inspectors and a new milk certification program. This, in turn, led to the creation of the Pure Food and Drug Act of 1906, a precursor to the Food and Drug Administration. This milk survey reinforced the foundation and institute's mission in the eyes of the public and embodied their goal of using science to solve public health issues. This was the first public health campaign undertaken by a Rockefeller institution.

The institute soon turned in a different direction, focusing solely on scientific research. The Rockefeller Institute Hospital opened in 1910 and served as the model for medical research centers that would follow in the coming decades.[13] Other major accomplishments included developing the vaccine for pneumococcal pneumonia, discovering DNA's purpose, developing a vaccine against yellow fever (accomplished by Max Theiler, working at the Rockefeller Foundation), and promoting modern-day cell biology. As for its primary direction into public health, soon other Rockefeller philanthropies were created to address these major public health issues. The institute has subsequently generated numerous Nobel Prizes.

Hookworm Eradication

In 1903, two years after the medical institute was created, Rockefeller Jr. started the General Education Board (GEB).[7] This organization was designed to improve education so that Southern farmers could improve productivity. Rockefeller Jr. founded the GEB after going on a train tour that focused on African American education in the South. The organization soon discovered that hookworm disease was raging there, causing problems for education and productive farming.

Hookworms are small worms that attach to the inside of the intestine. They live on small amounts of blood, but a heavy infection leads to anemia, which in turn causes weakness and debility. Eggs are excreted in the stool, then develop to a larval stage, which can penetrate the skin when picked up by a barefoot person. Warm rural areas of the South, where many people went barefoot, became an ideal place for the problem to take hold. Thus, not only people but also education and productive cash crops were affected.

Hookworm disease was unrecognized in the United States before being isolated in the early 20th century.[8,12] According to *ncpedia.org*, however, the disease had probably thrived for decades before that, brought to America by slaves from Africa.

Frederick Gates became interested in Stiles's research. Methods to diagnose and cure hookworm through quick fixes, such as collection of fecal samples, had been used during the occupation of Puerto Rico. These easy diagnosis methods appealed to Gates and Rockefeller. GEB had learned that building new schools in the South was not sufficient to alleviate poverty. Children who were infected with hookworm were malnourished and could not attend school. Infected adults could not be productive.[12] Both factors contributed to the cycle of poverty.

In 1909, Rockefeller established the Rockefeller Sanitary Commission for the Eradication of Hookworm Disease (abbreviated RSC) with $1 million. Charles Stiles persuaded Rockefeller to create this commission, stating that hookworm was one of the most important diseases of the South, causing the "proverbial laziness of the poorer white classes of the white population."[15] Although the RSC was intended to target a single disease, it helped to promote public health systems throughout the United States. The campaign highlighted the possibilities of public health work by eliminating a disease through dispensing of an anthelmintic drug, promoting shoe wearing and construction of latrines, and using public health propaganda.[9] During the five years of the RSC's existence, it treated approximately 700,000 people infected by hookworms.[15]

Wickliffe Rose, who was serving as dean of Peabody College at the time, was asked to become head of the RSC in 1910.[7] Rose saw hookworm as a means to prompt the government into strengthening public health systems. A professor by training, he believed that education was the key to solving public health issues. He wanted to focus on outreach and education. The RSC created demonstrations and public lectures with fanfare and festivity, attracting the public by allowing them to look through microscopes of organism samples, for example.

This campaign aimed to address the root causes of large issues that Gates had intended to address with philanthropy. The program did not fully eliminate the disease as intended. Hilton Head, South Carolina, still had hookworm in the 1960s, for example. (While homes for the rich were being built, workers often lived in trailers on muddy side streets.) Nevertheless, the effort did encourage the establishment of a public health infrastructure, such as county public health departments.[7] More than 1,370 counties in the South had full-time health directors by the time the RSC closed.

Moving Abroad: The International Health Commission (IHC)

Because of the successful work in the American South, the RSC prepared to extend its activities to other countries. While Rose was on
a trip to Egypt and Ceylon, however, Gates announced that the RSC
would be closed down in 1914.[15] Rose returned from his trip, conced-
ing that much more needed to be done, especially overseas. In January 1913, the *New York Times* published an article stating how crucial
the fight against hookworms was and urging that the campaign be extended abroad.[8] Consequently, in 1913, the board decided to create the
International Health Commission (IHC), which aimed to promote
"public sanitation and the spread of knowledge of scientific medicine."[16]
Unlike the RSC, the IHC undertook public health issues on a global
level. The Rockefeller Foundation believed that it could use its public
health successes from the American South and apply these methods internationally. Although the RSC closed down, its efforts against hookworm did not end. Its hookworm campaign extended first to the British
Empire, then to Latin America and Asia.[15]

The IHC collaborated with local governments, using specific diseases as the groundwork for larger public health projects, such as creating permanent public health agencies. The foundation believed that
it already possessed the domestic experience with health issues necessary to expand internationally. It recognized that improved public
health would lead to better sanitation and more productive societies.
This, in turn, would increase economic growth and decrease the likelihood of economic shocks, such as labor or socialist movements.[17] The
IHC also aimed to advance Western civilization through public health
campaigns in the developing world.[18] This public health division of
the foundation assumed different names as it changed course throughout its history; it was called the International Health Commission
from 1913 to 1916 and then the International Health Board from 1916
to 1927.

Wickliffe Rose was the first director of the IHC. As former director
of the RSC, he aimed to use the same tools of public awareness that

he had used in the American South for the new public health campaigns.[15] Rose operated the IHC as a copy of the RSC in its beginning years. He used hookworm disease as a means to several ends: courting local governments, raising awareness about public health, and urging governments to create and invest in their own public health systems. Rose believed that public health work was the responsibility of the government. He established that the IHC could help government agencies to organize their own public health campaigns by helping with financial resources and creating facilities for training public health professionals. He insisted that IHC aid be temporary—a position he eventually retracted so that governments could assume the costs and control.

All subsequent directors of the IHC held medical degrees, unlike Rose, which changed the course of its operations.[8] Frederick Russell, who succeeded Rose as director, promoted the discovery of new knowledge through research. He established laboratories in New York City to discover the paths of transmission of diseases. He built up the IHC to a higher level of professionalism and organization, and increased funding. Russell believed that public health tools and methods would lead to eradication of diseases. He believed that basic laboratory research was fundamental for public health campaigns.

Overall, all directors believed in certain key principles about the organization. First, they noted that philanthropy should not be confused with charity—philanthropy was an investment. It was meant to be given to governments,[12] not individuals. It was given in limited durations to limit dependence. The IHC believed that generating self-help was key, even if it had to withdraw funds when it did not see promise that recipients would continue the work.

By 1916, the IHC had extended its hookworm campaign to 15 different countries. Under Rose, it focused on outreach and education.[7] It aimed for local governments to take over the projects eventually, by initially urging them to take on the capital costs of the campaign.[6] Thus, governments assumed the costs of building latrines and sewage systems.

Soon, the IHC moved away from hookworm to other projects and campaigns. It had found that completely eradicating the disease would be unattainable for many countries. Hookworm disease was not eradicated, but the IHC had achieved its goal of creating a strong public health foundation for other public health diseases. The foundation had established key principles and methods for the fight against hookworms. Some of these principles included working jointly with local governments, conducting surveys of the infection, and creating a full outreach campaign for public health.

Among the other major diseases that the IHC soon turned to were yellow fever, malaria, and tuberculosis. Unlike most organizations today, the IHC operated behind the scenes, without the notice of the media or press.[9] It was careful to avoid campaigns that might be too time-consuming or costly, a lesson it learned after it became involved with tuberculosis in France during World War I. That disease had no magic bullets or easy technical solutions.[12] After that campaign, the IHC—realizing it was not a relief agency—vowed never again to become involved in such a lengthy campaign.[1] It subsequently ensured that each project was narrowly constructed so that its goals would be met every quarter in its reports. Each campaign was always carried out individually, which avoided tackling multiple causes at once. The IHC succeeded in transitioning its campaigns over to local governments by creating permanent government public health agencies.[12]

Public Health in an Age of Imperialism

During this age, philanthropy's role was uncertain, particularly in the arena of international philanthropy. Within the United States, the government and philanthropic actors worked hand in hand to provide social services. Other countries operated in different ways, with less private and philanthropic influence in providing social services to citizens.

Within global capitalism, the IHC rose to power, tackling the root causes of worker inefficiency, disease, and ill-health. It chose certain tropical diseases, such as malaria and yellow fever, because they impacted productivity. Philanthropy offered campaigns that aided market economies. By courting local governments with the public health campaigns, the foundation could enter the local country's system and gain political or economic influence for US corporations.[12] The foundation understood that the humanitarian nature of its campaigns also allowed it to create friendly international relations for the corporation. Although the Rockefeller Foundation, itself, was legally separate from Standard Oil, it often shared managers and trustees, particularly in the earlier years. The efforts of the IHC went well beyond increasing the well-being of populations.[12] It helped to stabilize colonies, spread Western cultural and bureaucratic standards, and prepare countries for foreign investments. Overall, the IHC's work helped to expand markets for global capitalism and stimulated economic growth for consumer markets.[15]

Yellow Fever

One of the most successful public health campaigns led by the Rockefeller Foundation was yellow fever control.[12] In 1898, when the United States was at the height of imperialism and commercial ascendance, it invaded Cuba. This permitted the expansion of control over the threat of yellow fever. The spread of this disease among the workers who completed the Panama Canal in 1914 had shown the deadliness of this virus. These factors prompted the Rockefeller Foundation to become interested in this disease.

The vector of yellow fever, *Aedes aegypti*, could survive aboard ships, thus spreading the virus through commercial ports. Ships going through the canal had to be quarantined, which caused long delays and extra costs. This practice disrupted trade and business, even though the disease killed a relatively small number of people.

Henry Rose Carter, an epidemiologist and expert in yellow fever, told Wickliffe Rose that he knew just what to do about yellow fever, that he could get rid of it in two years, and that "there is no uncertainty in it."[4] William Crawford Gorgas, a doctor who had helped to eradicate yellow fever in Cuba and the Panama Canal Zone, stated that its eradication would "command the attention and the gratitude of the world. And the thing can be done."[19]

Persuaded by these statements, the IHC established the Yellow Fever Commission in 1916. The foundation made Gorgas the head of that commission in South America. This commission succeeded in eliminating yellow fever in several countries, which led to additional campaigns across the world. A few years later, the Rockefeller Foundation hired Max Theiler, a South African scientist working at Harvard, to develop a vaccine. Theiler, working with virus samples isolated by a Rockefeller team in Nigeria, developed a vaccine, subsequently called 17D, based on a weaker form of the virus. Dr. A. J. Warren, assistant director of the IHC, was first given the vaccine. He did not display symptoms and produced blood that protected inoculated mice from the virus—proof that Theiler had created an effective vaccine. This vaccine was eventually used in World War II, when the US Army requested increased supplies of the vaccine. As a sign of patriotism, the Rockefeller Foundation donated the vaccines to the entire US military, free of charge.[16] To date, this 17D strain is the only vaccine used for yellow fever. Moreover, it is safe and effective. No other disease had such an impact on the Rockefeller Foundation's health division in all of its years. Yellow fever brought a new focus on laboratory work and medical research for the organization. And Theiler received a Nobel Prize for his accomplishment.

Malaria

From its inception, the IHC was interested in malaria, although unfamiliar with it. Wickliffe Rose had been introduced to mosquitos early in his career as IHC director during his interactions with Ronald Ross, the discoverer of the malaria mosquito life cycle.[8] Ross had initially worked in Hyderabad, India, the Liverpool School of Tropical Medicine, and then the London School of Hygiene and Tropical Medicine. He had received a Nobel Prize in Medicine, the first such prize for England.

Dr. Fred Soper acted as administrative head of the IHC's regional office during the yellow fever campaign. He steered the commission toward malaria after its success with yellow fever because he feared that once everyone was vaccinated for yellow fever, budgets for mosquito control would decline quickly. With the work on yellow fever, he was convinced that the eradication of mosquito vectors was possible. By this time, malaria was a major disease globally, and its high infection and fatality rates presented a good opportunity for the IHC to intervene. At the time, researchers and IHC officers were unsure of how to tackle the disease. Some preferred campaigns against the larvae; others regarded treatment with quinine a more effective method.

In 1917, the IHC began a campaign closer to home, in Mississippi and Arkansas, where different methods were tested. In one county, mosquito-breeding grounds were eliminated through drainage techniques. Elsewhere, screens were installed in windows. In other counties, the commission distributed quinine to those infected with malaria. The IHC also tried using quinine as a preventive medicine. Its goal was to discover which method would be best to control malaria in the temperate American southern climate. These campaigns, designed to eliminate mosquitos in general, were also instrumental in creating county health units to educate the public about health and sanitation. The foundation's president at the time, George Vincent, stated that, "malaria eradication is feasible, scientifically and economically. It represents a striking contribution to community progress and human happiness."[8]

By the 1920s, the IHC had expanded its malaria campaign to Nicaragua, Puerto Rico, and Brazil. Soon, the commission started to use a newly discovered method of mosquito eradication, Paris Green. A combination of copper acetate, arsenic trioxide, and road dust, this form of mosquito control was called species sanitation. Unlike previous methods, in which mosquito eradication in cities and quinine distribution in rural areas were used, this practice was feasible in both rural and urban situations. By 1928, the IHC had expanded its campaigns to more than 20 countries overseas. During World War II, it discovered the impact of DDT, which seemed to have completely revolutionized the field of malaria control.[12] In 1940, the IHC eliminated *Anopheles gambiae*, a species that spread malaria in Brazil. The

Rockefeller Foundation remained dedicated to the fight against malaria into its later years, helping to create public–private partnerships for malaria in Africa in the late 1990s.

The New Global Health Scene

Before the World Health Organization (WHO) was founded in 1948, the IHC was the world's most significant public health agency.[8] In the first half of the 20th century, most international health efforts relied on private organizations. The League of Nations Health Organization (LNHO) was the main intergovernmental health body at the time; it depended heavily on the Rockefeller Foundation.[20] The LNHO, founded after World War I, was modeled after the Rockefeller's IHC. The Rockefeller Foundation saw the LNHO as a means for advancing its goals of raising overall health globally through the growth of scientific and medical knowledge. The foundation not only helped create the LNHO, but it also supported it and then revived it after World War II.

By the 1950s, many organizations were focused on natural sciences, prompting the Rockefeller Foundation to disband its biology division in 1951. World War II brought on complications, such as refugees, food shortages, and epidemics. With the end of the war and new health concerns for its population, the United States increased its government funding for health initiatives and multilateral organizations.[17]

WHO's founding led to the closing of the IHC. Although the IHC disbanded, the Rockefeller Foundation still maintained an indirect presence in the public health field.[8] For instance, IHC's former employees helped to staff WHO. Unlike the IHC, WHO had more universal membership and it was better funded than the LNHO. However, the IHC's methods, values, and organizational style permeated the infrastructure of WHO.[12] When the IHC closed, it was in an era of belief in the efficacy of biomedical methods to improve health. The biomedical perspective that the IHC had spread rose to prominence in the international health agenda. Its influence did not end, as WHO's Global Malaria Eradication Program was largely staffed by former IHC employees.[17]

Spreading the Public Health Gospel

The Rockefeller Foundation left basic principles of global health that have permeated our methods of disease control, institutionalization of agencies, and cooperation with local governments.[12] Today, we see a type of public health perspective of work that concentrates on research, biomedical approaches, and technical solutions. In 1960, WHO's Expert Committee on Malaria stated that any malaria-eradication program would need to be developed along with health services;[8] this stance would have pleased Rose, who had instilled this belief in the creation of long-term local public health services within the IHC's programs. WHO soon used malaria as an incentive for developing rural health services, much like the RSC or IHC had used hookworm to develop public health departments globally.[17]

The foundation has undoubtedly left its mark on the world of public health in many ways.[12] The disease-centered approach it used can still be traced through many public health institutions today. During the first part of the 20th century, in particular, support for the germ theory and for science and technology as the answers for social ills were popular.[1] The Rockefeller Foundation pioneered international health by providing the groundwork for a new health strategy with its own type of bureaucracy.[12] It helped to popularize public health through the creation of national public health departments throughout the world. It not only generated political and public support for public health, but it also advocated for the institutionalization of international health.[21,22]

The IHC was unique for its time because it operated as a philanthropic organization but also as a national, bilateral, multilateral, and transnational agency when no other such agencies existed. The foundation used budget incentives by encouraging the national government to assume the costs of the public health campaigns. The government would take over between 20% and 100% of the costs of the campaigns in just a few years. Thus, the foundation's self-defined measure of success—that it would generate national support for public health in each of its operating districts—was met.[15] Indeed, it set the agenda for a new type of philanthropy and public health activity that other organizations would soon follow.[17] The foundation's success was made possible by its officers' extensive training and their local engagement. Its techniques in disease control, coupled with government cooperation, enabled the foundation to instill a belief in public health throughout the world.[8] The foundation's ultimate indicator of success was that it was able to sustain the institutionalization of public health.

The Rockefeller Foundation was the wealthiest philanthropic entity in its time, which allowed it to gain its level of power.[8] Before the IHC was created in 1913, the Rockefeller name was associated with unimaginable power, corruption, and evil capitalism.[8] The role of the IHC was crucial in improving the Rockefeller image. But it also helped to improve the health of the people it was targeting and stimulated the institutionalization of schools of public health, since the foundation's programs required trained personnel. The foundation left basic principles of global health that have permeated our methods of disease control, institutionalization of agencies, and cooperation with local governments.[12]

Concluding Thoughts
BILL FOEGE

At the beginning of the 20th century, the Rockefeller Foundation pioneered the growth and power of public health. A century later, the Bill & Melinda Gates Foundation provided the tipping point for global health. In both cases, these foundations brought resources to underfunded needs, changing what governments needed to do to protect the health of their citizens. The Rockefeller Foundation forced people to raise their sights to see what could be accomplished if science was exploited. Science gets its power by being used, not just existing. The Gates Foundation forced global health people to stop thinking like poor people and raise their sights to what is needed to actually change health globally. Global health equity became the ultimate objective of all public health activities.

CHAPTER 12

The New Philanthropy

KIERA CHAN

The tipping point for global health occurred at the turn of the 21st century, when the Gates family became interested in the subject. In the 1900s, the topic was a minor subject in schools of public health or medicine. Today, the interest in global health is apparent in every school of higher learning in much of the world.

It was not just the sheer power and size of the Bill & Melinda Gates Foundation that jumpstarted a new century of global health. It was also the approach that Bill and Melinda took to the subject. They thoroughly researched the subject and supported research aimed at poor people in poor countries.[1] They provided pathways for students to enter the field. They visited public health leaders and politicians to smooth over conflicting interests and to create partnerships to make global health decisions more unified.[2] And they sought the advice of Bill Gates Sr., a lawyer, to help organize a response to the problems that were denying the benefit of science to so many people of limited income. Bill and Melinda then visited the homes of people in low-income countries, staying overnight in African villages; they became schooled in how science and technology could aid them. And in the process, the foundation ushered in a new century of global health.[3]

Over the last two decades, the size of the philanthropic sector has grown significantly.[4] Today, there are more than 200,000 foundations in the world; 86,000 are registered in the United States. With the Gates Foundation leading the way, more foundations are investing in global health. But how did the philanthropic foundation sector become so large, with such a significant role, especially in global health?

Before the 1900s, philanthropy was nascent, mostly consisting of charity to those in need in local areas. Then, in the 1910s, Andrew Carnegie and John D. Rockefeller entered the field, creating a new name for philanthropy—scientific giving—with their subsequent foundations.[5] In the 1950s, the Ford Foundation became the first billion-dollar foundation.

Before 2000—almost precisely 100 years after the Rockefeller Foundation shaped the world of international health, founding early public health institutions, academic institutions, and formal health partnerships—the Gates Foundation entered the philanthropic world, changing the face of global health for the future.[6,7] In June 2006, Warren E. Buffett pledged over $30 billion to the Gates Foundation.[6] In 2020, Wikipedia listed it as the second most well-funded foundation in the world.

Both the Rockefeller and Gates Foundations entered the public health scene at critical points: Rockefeller, when global health was barely in existence; the Gates Foundation, when global health was limping along. Although both foundations have faced many criticisms as global health pioneers, their contributions to spur the field with resources, innovation, leadership, and motivation helped set the trends for the future of global health.

Rockefeller's foundation was begun in 1913 to "search for a cause, an attempt to cure evils at their source."[8] Without it, as we reported in the chapter on early philosophy (chapter 11), the institutionalization of public health agencies such as the World Health Organization (WHO) might not have transpired. That foundation's International Health Division, for example, helped to instill the ideas of public health and to formalize health institutions.[8] And former International Health Division employees even helped to staff and start up WHO.

Setting the Stage for the Gates Foundation

With the rise of globalization and the subsequent new health threats that accompanied it, a more coordinated global approach was needed. Multilateral agencies provided an important step, but the funding of WHO was inadequate to meet the world's needs.

Oil shocks and other economic crises in the 1970s and 1980s led to decreased donor funding to WHO. The Ronald Reagan administration froze US funding to the organization in the 1980s to formally reprimand WHO for a series of anti-US corporate-funding policies and programs. When the Cold War ended, Western bloc support of WHO declined, and Cold War spending for international health dissipated. Some even questioned whether WHO was needed. Global health workers often adopted the mentality of the poor: that resources would not improve and that the emphasis should be on "making do" with inadequate funds, rather than thinking boldly about what needed to be done.

Often, such apathy spread to the global health community itself. Differences of opinion inhibited efficient work rather than stimulating discussion for better approaches. One point of contention was whether global health problems should be addressed horizontally or vertically. An example of the former is WHO's strategy, following an important conference in Alma-Ata in 1978, when it called for strengthening the infrastructure. UNICEF, on the other hand, adopted an approach of concentrating on specific interventions that could improve health immediately for some. This led to a program called GOBI (Growth monitoring, Oral rehydration, Breastfeeding, and Immunizations)—a vertical approach.[6,9] In the United States, health programs improved with a combination of vertical and horizontal efforts. Every new tool was exploited, which improved the infrastructure and led to rapid incorporation of the next tool. Horizontal and vertical efforts alternated in ratcheting up health programs.

The insight that both approaches were necessary led to private philanthropy's aid to efforts that would have historically been under the government's mantle. Funds for mass vaccination in low-income countries were inadequate, and overall funding for global health seemed to be at a low point.[9] But then, in the 1980s, immunization levels in the world increased greatly as foundations, governments, and industry supported a global effort to improve childhood immunization, under a plan developed by the Task Force for Child Survival. Then, even *that* progress disintegrated when leaders of UNICEF and WHO were replaced.[7]

The History of Gavi

The Gates Foundation turned this situation around, stepping in with a $750 million, five-year grant to establish the Global Alliance for Vaccines and Immunization (Gavi) in 1999.[4] This hybrid organization facilitates the work of WHO and UNICEF, combining foundation, government, corporations, and others into a global approach.

Ever since the inception of their foundation, Bill and Melinda Gates have been interested in areas that received inadequate attention and were underfunded.[1] They learned that vaccines developed in the United States took many years to reach the people in low-income settings who really needed them. They learned that millions of children die every year from preventable diseases.[10] The Gateses realized that the value of a child in the developing world was not weighted the same as a child in the developed world. After seeing the statistics and hearing these stories countless times, they decided to take action.

Bringing a vaccine to market usually costs almost $900 million. The cost of establishing new vaccines discourages many from producing vaccines for poor countries.[8] But the Gates Foundation could leverage its power to bring the National Institutes of Health, pharmaceutical companies, scientific researchers, and corporate product developers together in a formal partnership.[11,12] In 1999, representatives from the vaccine industry, global health bilateral agencies, and UN agencies came together to form GAVI (now Gavi)[13]—facilitated by the Gates Foundation grant mentioned earlier. This alliance was able to reduce prices significantly by purchasing in bulk or buying underused vaccines.

The Gates Foundation helped to subsidize the purchase of newer vaccines. It also funded clinical trials to help bring new vaccines to market, particularly the market for lower-income countries.[14] The foundation was able to use market incentives to save lives. The fund stimulated vaccine development through "push" mechanisms, while rewarding countries for delivering vaccines through "pull" mechanisms.* This global partnership helped to coordinate efforts throughout all stages of vaccination, including development, production, and delivery.

Since 2000, the funding for WHO has increased due to international philanthropy's work with UN agencies. Now, the Gates Foundation is the single largest contributor to WHO, after the United States.[7]

The Gavi partnership has had far-reaching impact beyond bringing vaccinations to children in the developing world. It helped to increase trust among the public, WHO, and pharmaceutical companies.[12] It also established a global market for high-quality, lower-priced vaccines—a market that had not previously existed.[6] The foundation also helped to renew global health's commitment toward immunization.[14] This organization established a model for a new type of partnership, the Global Public Private Partnership.[13] Later, Gavi was used as a standard to develop other organizations and partnerships, such as the Global Fund (to fight HIV/AIDS, TB, and malaria).

A Change in Strategy

In 2005, the World Health Assembly invited Bill Gates to address its 58th assembly.[15,16] This was only the second time that someone from

---

* Push programs included creating tax credits for research and development to subsidize the costs. Pull programs included creating patent outputs or advance-purchase commitments to reward research and development. Push mechanisms have been instrumental in stimulating development of products in the early stages of research, while pull mechanisms help to bind companies into commitments towards specific diseases and research.[1]

the private sector had addressed the assembly. (Bill Foege was the first, five years earlier.) Gates's speech centered around the importance of vaccination and disease eradication. He recalled that smallpox was eradicated with the aid of technology and vaccinations. He suggested that the next success in public health should also invoke such interventions. His speech was important because it helped to orient the path of global health and its priorities toward vaccination and technological solutions.

Six years later, in 2011, Bill Gates was asked to produce and present a report at the G20 Summit in Cannes, France.[17] Gates advocated three goals: (1) to focus on direct outcomes that would contribute to the Millennium Development Goals, (2) to provide real-time data around programs for anyone to access, and (3) to increase evaluation of programs for development. The foundation became more involved in powerful partnerships in global health as well as policy and decision-making. It was also able to help set the course of global health priorities, as this summit illustrates, and to establish norms around global health development.[7] All these factors, in turn, contributed to an increase in power and legitimacy for the foundation.

The Gates Foundation also prides itself on its Intellectual Ventures Laboratory, which creates new and affordable technologies for health. By forming sustainable business partnerships and investing, this laboratory minimizes business risk and attracts scientific innovators.

As illustrated by Gavi, the Gates Foundation creates unique and sustainable partnerships. It also aids and spurs on existing ones.[18] During the Gates Foundation's polio-eradication efforts in Nigeria, there was heightened skepticism about the partnerships and mistrust among the government and the donors.[2] The government believed that Westerners might be contaminating the vaccines with HIV, and, as a result, did not want to become involved with the eradication program. To smooth out these conflicts, Bill Gates visited and created formal agreements to commit the Gates Foundation to the program.

In other partnerships, the foundation set up the host country with the tools for success and slowly turned over the program to the country. The China–Gavi vaccine program, for example, built upon China's existing vaccination efforts, helped to increase vaccine coverage in rural China, and introduced new mechanisms such as using auto-disable syringes.[14] The program has graduated from its support from the Gates Foundation, proving the sustainability of its methods.

Shifting into Other Areas of Health

Starting with a goal of decreasing child mortality in developing countries, programs spread to other areas, such as women's empowerment. Melinda Gates traveled the world for the foundation's activities and listened to the plight of women and their stories.[16] The women kept telling her that they wished they had the ability to choose when to have children, to have access to contraceptives, to go to school, and to earn an income. They told her that they didn't want more children because they couldn't afford to feed the ones they already had.

She asked public advocates for women's issues what her foundation could do to help. They said that the best way to support public advocates was for her to become one, so she did. As the foundation became more involved in women's empowerment, maternal and child health, and family planning, Melinda realized that investing in women was the greatest investment because it leads to investing in their families and society overall. The foundation decided to take on a large role in women's issues.

In 2003, the Bill & Melinda Gates Foundation announced its "Grand Challenges in Global Health Initiative," which encouraged researchers to carry out "unorthodox" projects.[7] The foundation pledged over $200 million for grants in the initial startup of the program for scientists to research diseases that were usually neglected.[8] This program led the foundation to become the largest donor in research for diseases in low-income countries.[1]

Ten years after the launch of the program, approaches changed when it could not effectively research or implement projects without strengthening health systems. It encountered several hurdles. For example, to improve sanitation in the slums of India, the foundation tried importing high-tech toilets; it was not a practical solution.[19] However, the foundation changed to meet the needs of its beneficiaries.

Investment in global health issues encouraged other private actors, such as foundations and public state actors, to invest in these areas as well. One notable partnership was the African Comprehensive HIV/AIDS Partnership (ACHAP).[8] It included the Gates Foundation, the government of Botswana, and Merck Pharmaceuticals, with input from Harvard University, USAID, and others. In less than five years, HIV-positivity rates for newborns dropped from 40% to 4%, proof that 21st-century science can be applied under African conditions.

In 2010, the Gateses and Warren Buffett instituted the "Giving Pledge," in which over 158 millionaires committed to spend much of their wealth in philanthropy.[4] The foundation has increased funding not only in AIDS research but also in global health overall. The National Institutes of Health, following the Gates Foundation lead, has increased its own spending on global health by $1 billion.[8]

Criticism, of course, abounds. *The Lancet* once doubted the foundation's future plans, stating that

> it is hard to know for sure. The first guiding principle of the Foundation is that it is "driven by the interests and passions of the Gates family." An annual letter from Bill Gates summarizes those passions, referring to newspapers, articles, books, and chance events that have shaped the Foundation's strategy. For such a large and influential investor in global health, is such a whimsical governance principle good enough?[20]

However, in 2015, Bill, anticipating a pandemic, said in a TedTalk that, "If anything kills over 10 million people in the next few decades, it's most likely to be a highly infectious virus rather than a war. Not missiles, but microbes."[21] He stated that many other countries barely invest in global health to stop a pandemic and that the world would not be prepared for a future pandemic. Gates noted that a virus much like the Spanish flu of 1918 would sweep across the globe, killing millions.[22] As a result, investments of the Gates Foundation were aimed at helping the world to prepare for a pandemic.

Philanthropy has also been able to target controversial or large-scale issues that were difficult for governments to address. These have included the vaccine crisis, sexual reproductive health issues, and family planning.

A repeated criticism is that WHO and state actors are accountable to donors and recipients but that foundations are only accountable for themselves.[22] However, foundations are attempting to be transparent by making information on activities and decisions freely available to all.[5]

Foundations will remain powerful global health actors. The Gates Foundation has been the subject of this chapter, but it is now one of dozens of foundations changing the potential of the world to reach an objective of global health equity.

Personal View of Philanthropy

BILL FOEGE

Among the great experiences in my career has been the ability to watch philanthropy up close. My first such encounter was to serve on the board for a small foundation, the Wheat Ridge Foundation. It provided resources domestically and globally for health, education, and social improvements.

This was followed by board membership on the MacArthur Foundation, where I was impressed by the care shown to fund projects in many fields of health, education, and justice, together with grants to meet the needs of Chicago, where that foundation is located. The quality of the staff, board discussions, careful study by board members, and constant desire to evaluate the results of its programs made it clear the board could be trusted with the endowment that made the foundation possible. Its program to identify exceptional people and provide them with a sizeable fellowship, with no strings attached, was unique. In talking to past MacArthur Fellows, they often said that recognition had allowed them freedom and status that led them to do much more in their field.

Membership on the Rockefeller Board was an honor because of its pioneering and continuing work in global health. As mentioned elsewhere, in many ways the Rockefeller health staff helped to launch WHO. While I was on the board, it approved unconventional activities, such as providing resources to the new director of WHO, Gro Brundtland, to use for unrestricted activities. She hired some exceptional people to take WHO into new and important areas. It approved money for a program to seek a vaccine for AIDS and persuaded one of its own, Dr. Seth Berkley, to head the program. This inspired the Gates Foundation to support the same program. The Rockefeller Foundation hosted many watershed global health meetings at its property in Bellagio, Italy.

Membership on the Hilton Foundation Board was yet another great learning experience. It funded global projects, such as village water systems in Africa, but also had domestic programs to meet the problems of homelessness. Conrad Hilton had enormous gratitude for the Catholic Sisters, who had helped him as a child. (Catholic Sisters is a global network of 700,000 vowed women religious around the world. In America, the Sisters have played a major role in education, nursing, and social work since the early 19th century.) The foundation provides substantial support to Sisters' programs. Anyone who has worked on the ground knows the efficiency and effectiveness of those programs. The foundation also provides a humanitarian award each year. Having been on various award juries over the years, I have never seen a program this exhaustive. Each year several hundred programs are reviewed, and about 20 are selected for jury decisions. Extensive material on each of the 20 is reviewed by the jury as its members debate, ask questions of the staff, and, finally, make a selection. To get a Hilton Humanitarian Prize is to receive the Nobel Prize in the humanitarian field.

The Marguerite Casey Foundation was created in this century. The seed was work done by other Casey entities for foster children. The new foundation concentrates on prevention, with results that will extend to future generations. Programs to give power to local organizations, grassroot efforts, and support for young people brought the board to disenfranchised communities around the country. To witness previously silent people find their voices, actually visit their congresspersons, and give talks to organizations was heartening. Inspired young people give power to other young people.

Finally, my years working at the Gates Foundation, starting in 1999, led to a profound respect for what passion, empathy, resources, talent, and leadership can do for global health. The early years were characterized by a thirst for knowledge on global health. At one point, Bill and Melinda sent a request for some books on global health. An inquiry to their staff offered no clue on the number of books I should send, but the answer did include the phrase, "Do not underestimate them." I sent emails to people in the field, asking which one or two publications would they most like the Gates to read. Some weeks later, staff went to Microsoft to deliver boxes containing 82 books.

Weeks later, I asked Bill if he had been able to look at any of them, and he said he had read 17 already. I asked what was the best one so far, and he said the 1993 World Bank Report, which included the concept of disability-adjusted life years (DALYs). He went on to explain his great interest in the concept and his discomfort with some parts of the equations used. The use of DALYs allows one to combine morbidity and mortality in a single number, thereby allowing the comparison of the burden of diseases with different mortality figures and also comparisons of such factors as regions and genders. The interest of the Gates family and their diligence in pursuing solutions did indeed inspire the tipping point for all of global health.

Concluding Thoughts

BILL FOEGE

This chapter concentrated mainly on US philanthropic organizations and thus is derelict in not pointing out the growth of philanthropy in other countries. Philanthropic organizations in Africa, Mexico, and India come readily to mind.

However, the failure to discuss the Novo Nordisk Foundation, the world's largest foundation, located in Denmark and focused on biomedical and biotechnology research, and the Wellcome Trust, in the United Kingdom, which supports science to "solve the urgent health challenges facing everyone," are major oversights. The author hopes for additional years to correct these omissions in a second edition.

It is true that foundations can make decisions in the absence of official public approval. The worst ones can use that advantage for promoting unsafe activities and policies. The best ones are aware of this advantage and seek transparency and feedback.

On the positive side, philanthropy has been of extreme importance in supporting early education programs, researching scientific questions, and even developing drugs and vaccines.

The net conclusion is one of great gratitude for philanthropy by the global health community.

CHAPTER 13

Pharmaco-Philanthropy and Global Health

BILL FOEGE

Pharmaceutical companies have always had programs to provide medications for those unable to pay, differential pricing for poor countries, and charitable donations. But it is only in the past 40 years that major programs have been developed for income-poor countries, often in connection with foundations or government agencies. Philanthropy from these corporations now provides a significant ingredient in global health programs. Below are some examples.

River Blindness (Onchocerciasis)

A farmer feels the sharp bite of a blackfly, an immediate annoyance, but she has no idea it will lead to a bleak final chapter of blindness. African farmers have tilled the land for generations without recognizing that the blindness of the village elders, often starting in their 40s, is related to the location of their farms. The soil is fertile, located near the river, and yields good crops; but the price is high near fast-flowing rivers and streams, where the *Simulium* flies breed. As they bite, they extract microfilaria of a parasite called Onchocerca. The microfilaria develop through a stage in the fly and return to humans during a subsequent blood meal. The new stage evolves into an adult in the human and begins to produce numerous microfilaria, to continue the cycle.

After multiple bites, the thousands of microfilariae that course through the body cause problems. The worst is blindness, which develops over a period of years as the microfilaria migrate through the eye. But these microfilaria also cause itching as they infiltrate the skin. Unfortunately, the adult parasite lives an average of a dozen years, and so it can bombard the body with microfilaria for an extended period. Multiple adult worms compound the problem.

In villages near these fast-flowing streams, it is common for children to become guides for their blind elders, often being at the leading edge of a stick, guiding the person. The life expectancy of rural Africans with blindness tends to be very short. It can be a bleak existence.

Merck

Into this sad scene, a corporation unexpectedly provided hope. The Merck Drug Company received a soil sample from a Japanese golf course; analysis of the sample showed an organism, *Streptomyces avermitilis*, and from this Merck developed a chemical the company named Ivermectin. It had a significant impact on heartworms in dogs and soon became the standard treatment for preventing that disease. Heartworms are caused by a parasitic worm called *Dirofilaria immitis*, transmitted by mosquitoes. Ivermectin, given once a month, can prevent the disease, and it was soon marketed under the name HeartGard.

Bill Campbell at Merck wondered if the drug might be of use with human parasites, and he talked to Roy Vagelos, head of research at Merck, about testing it in Africa. Merck realized that the drug would have a limited market, but Vagelos provided the resources, and a Merck scientist, Mohammad Aziz, began the African trials.

In February 1981, the first human tests were conducted at the University of Dakar. By 1983, the results were so encouraging that Phase 2 studies began. By 1986, Phase 3 studies on 1,200 patients in Ghana and Liberia were completed, demonstrating the impact of the drug as well as the optimal dosing.

The drug was found to kill the microfilaria of *Onchocerca* organisms. In fact, it was even more efficient against this human parasite than against heartworms in dogs. Given once a year, Ivermectin not only killed microfilariae but also prevented production of additional microfilariae for about a year. The drug did not kill the adult female worms, but it did render them temporarily sterile. In 1987, papers were filed in France for regulatory approval of Ivermectin, marketed as Mectizan.

Clearly, profits would be limited. An inexpensive drug, given only once a year to some of the poorest people in the world, would yield small returns on investment. By this time, Roy Vagelos had become the CEO of Merck, and the company decided to donate the drug. But how could this work? On October 21, 1987, at press conferences in Washington, DC, and Paris, Merck announced that it would supply Mectizan, for the treatment of river blindness, to everyone who needed it, for as long as necessary, at no charge.

Merck offered the drug to the World Health Organization (WHO), only to be stymied by its bureaucracy. Merck next went to the US Agency for International Development (USAID), again offering the drug free if that agency would develop a system of distribution. USAID said it was not interested. Years later, the person who directed USAID at the time explained the disinterest by saying that the agency was "simply too busy."

Merck was dismayed by this lack of interest but tried yet again. On December 17, 1987, the company sent John Lyons and Jerry Jackson to visit with the Task Force for Child Survival in Atlanta, Georgia, to make the same offer it had presented to WHO and USAID. The task force was interested but expressed several concerns. How long would the offer of free Ivermectin actually continue? Merck said that, for human use with river blindness, it would be offered for as long as needed. The other major concern revolved around potential adverse effects when the drug was given to millions of people. The plan of execution therefore started cautiously. Surveillance of villages was conducted for 72 hours after drug distribution to monitor adverse reactions. The surveillance period was subsequently reduced to 48 hours, then 24 hours, and then abandoned. It is one of the safest drugs known at the low doses used in the program.*

What is the background of Merck that would suggest such a socially conscious move? History is always a book opened in the middle, but we must begin someplace. In 1668, Friedrich Jacob Merck bought a drug store in Darmstadt, Germany. The Merck Company was born. In 1891, George Merck came to the United States and started Merck and Co.

Reconstructing the ethos of this company is difficult, but George Merck once declared, "We try never to forget that medicine is for the people. It is not for profits. And if we have remembered that, they have never failed to appear." Add Roy Vagelos to that philosophy and you understand what followed.

Attempts at Controlling the Parasite

Onchocerciasis, the disease, was first described in 1893. The life cycle was finally understood in 1926. In 1974, a massive program was initiated in West Africa by WHO, the United Nations Development Programme, the Food and Agriculture Organization, and the World Bank. The program was based on helicopters or fixed-wing aircrafts spraying insecticides in streams and rivers to kill the blackfly larvae, the vector of the parasite.

The program was very successful in the countries that participated. But a major problem was that Nigeria was excluded. That country was recovering from a destructive civil war, and participating agencies were unwilling to become involved, fearing the country's instability. But Nigeria harbored some of the largest river blindness areas in Africa.

---

* However, it is not for sale for human use in the United States, and unfortunately, some people have used Ivermectin for the prevention of coronavirus, using the animal formulations and in doses much higher than used for onchocerciasis. Even safe drugs can become a hazard when misused.

Mectizan now provided another approach to controlling the disease. With a free drug available, mechanisms had to be developed to get the drug to the right people in the correct dosage. The inability of WHO to provide a plan had seemed devastating at the beginning, but it became a blessing in that it forced new thinking on how to deliver global health. A small group from Merck and the task force thought through the issues.

First, the decision about who should get the drug led to the conclusion that it should be easily obtained by organizations working in rural areas of Africa. These included mission groups and nongovernmental organizations, but also a growing number of government health programs. A form was developed that encouraged applicants to tell how they would distribute the drug to the right people in the correct dosage, keep records on who had received the drug and when, note any adverse reactions, and document how they would secure the drug so it did not end up in the markets for use on animals. The applicants also were encouraged to make this distribution of Mectizan an annual event. In this way, it was hoped that microfilaria could be reduced until adult worms in humans had died. The application form had to be submitted through the ministry of health. This step kept the ministry abreast of such activities, promoted the cooperation of health programs with the government, and provided the ministry with the opportunity to become actively involved.

A group at the task force studied the applications and made recommendations to the Expert Committee on Mectizan. This committee was financially supported by Merck but was independent. Merck had nonvoting members on the committee to improve transparency, and every effort was made to fill all requests that met the guidelines. Decisions did not require the input of any global agency, and Merck avoided having to make the distribution decisions. It became an early example, as was the Task Force for Child Survival, of organizations that constituted the mortar between the bricks of the global agencies. These mortar groups made the global agencies better. (See chapter 10 on hybrid organizations.) Soon, WHO sought a role that was much more useful than if it had been in charge of the program.

Results were far better than anyone expected. The safety of the drug encouraged more groups to request participation. The drug itself provided marketing opportunities not anticipated. Ivermectin also proved virtually 100% effective against roundworms and whipworms. People were pleased to be treated for roundworms. But, even more dramatic, for many people, was the relief they experienced from the disease's intense itching. Many experienced the first day they could recall without incessant itching. Some had suffered for years with itching being the first thing they knew in the morning and the last thing they knew at night. Now that was gone. And they told others.

Soon President Carter became involved in urging heads of state in Africa to join the effort. Along with Roy Vagelos, CEO of Merck, Carter visited areas with high blindness rates. The combination of reduced itching at the local level and the efforts of Vagelos and Carter at the highest government levels made marketing success inevitable. The early goal of reaching 6 million people in six years was reached in only four years. And then success bred success. The World Bank developed a fund to help in the distribution of Mectizan, making it easier for even underfunded health efforts to develop programs.

Innovations also developed at the field level. Instead of weighing people to determine dosage, a measuring stick was developed, and height was used to determine the right amount of Mectizan to dispense. A line at a certain height on the stick indicated that the person should get a single tablet; a higher level required 1½ tablets; above a certain height, the person would get 2 tablets. This simple tool worked because of the drug's great safety margins.

Originally, operations were conducted by a mobile team, but with experience it was found that a villager could safely conduct the operation. Villagers were so pleased with the results of treatment that they would name a trusted person, such as a schoolteacher or religious leader, to be the person in charge. Records were kept, and visits by health workers allowed a review of the completeness of the program.

A typical experience was recorded by an outside evaluation team on November 4, 1997, at a village in Mali. The group included visiting Merck employees and a gathering of village leaders. One bench was devoted to blind people, who told their stories to the evaluation team. One young man, only 39 years of age, had been blind for 21 years. Blind for over half of his life!

The people in that village were very sophisticated about onchocerciasis. They knew that their children would never have to put up with this cause of blindness, and they were grateful. The visit helped Merck employees see the impact of their efforts. But it was also a chance for the villagers to become connected, to see Merck employees, and to know that medicine doesn't just appear in a village by magic. They saw the faces of people who spend their days worrying about schedules and customs, about dosage and packaging, about storage and records. It takes the whole world to raise a healthy child!

The economist John Maynard Keynes once said, "The day is not far off when economic problems will take a back seat to our real problems." He was talking about human relations, about creativity, behavior, health, and religion. Maybe October 21, 1987, the day of the Merck announcement that the company would give Mectizan free, was that day—the moment when a corporation had the audacity to make social need more important than profits. To make a commitment that went beyond what could actually be seen. To treat anyone free, as long as required.

Are there precedents? There are a few. Wyeth Pharmaceuticals provided the patent for bifurcated needles to WHO. Tata Industries took responsibility for smallpox eradication in parts of Bihar, India. But Merck took corporate philanthropy to a new level and started a growing trend in global health. The market has its rules. When there is a problem, who will win? The marketplace, of course.

In this case, however, the management team at Merck decided social need would win. Relook at the commitment. Not as long as Mectizan paid its way through sales of HeartGard in the United States. Not as long as it fit into their plan. "As long as needed for the treatment of onchocerciasis." Forever, if necessary.

But Merck also benefited. At a time when company loyalty is often of secondary importance to those seeking higher wages, it became

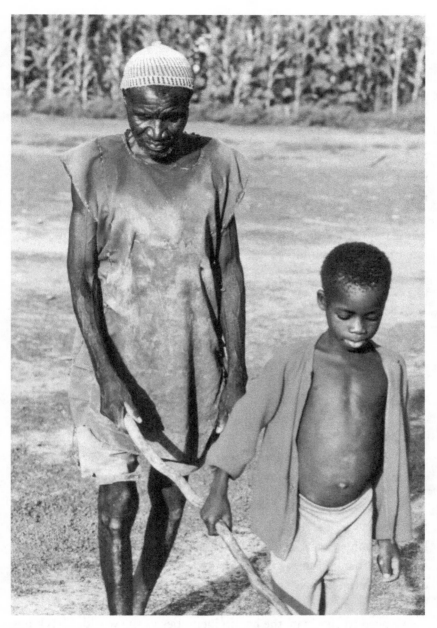

This iconic image of a child leading a blind elder will soon be known by history only. Because of Mectizan, river blindness has reached such low levels that the morbidity caused by the disease, particularly visual impairment and blindness, is no longer prevalent.
Source: US Agency for International Development/DVIDS, US Department of Defense/Science Photo Library.

apparent that workers like being associated with a company interested in social benefits. It is hard to put a value on this kind of benefit, but it helps to retain good people.

There are other lessons. One is the miracle of coalitions. It started quite small with a few people on the Mectizan expert committee, the group interested at Merck, and the Onchocerciasis Control Program in West Africa. But it grew. As mission groups found they could get Mectizan—but only if they applied through the ministry of health to the committee—the coalition widened. Soon even the World Bank was involved in developing a fund for distributing Mectizan.

At this point, the program was reaching 20 million people a year. But it required a coalition chain that would continue to grow. Every one of those 20 million people was at the end of a line that included

- Applications requiring mail, telephone, fax, and computers
- A secretariat and committee
- Orders placed and sorted in New Jersey
- Tablets bottled, boxed, and shipped from France
- Airlines and customs, clearance and ministries, storage and delivery
- A pipeline that branched into thousands of spigots
- Clinics, mobile teams, village workers, drivers, enumerators, and scribes
- Dirt roads, flooded rivers, war and conflict, and every ample barrier that Africa has to offer in reaching its poor

Despite the odds, it actually worked. We can never become too jaded to simply accept that such programs actually work to improve the health of someone beyond the usual health system. Soon a decrease in disease transmission was documented, and it was even possible to dream of a time when onchocerciasis would be a memory, a footnote in medical texts, a curiosity in the oral history of a village.

We need to eliminate the health inequities of the world. Merck has used its scientific capacity to go beyond profit to provide a significant social benefit to a population that would not otherwise benefit. Merck has targeted an inequity.

A second challenge is to promote the positive benefits of globalism. Villagers forgotten by their own health ministries were now benefiting from sophisticated research, transportation, and communications, thanks to developments in other countries.

A third need is to use the resources of today for the benefit of generations yet to come. Much of our exploitation has actually borrowed from the future. The Mectizan program changes the future: the deeds of today also meet the needs of tomorrow.

The impact of this program is being recognized. There is a metal sculpture, *Sightless among Miracles* by R. T. "Skip" Walker, that was commissioned by John Moores, one of the outstanding warriors in the battle against onchocerciasis. The sculpture shows the familiar figure of a small boy, investing in the future of his African village by using a stick to guide a blind man. The first copy of this sculpture was dedicated in the Merck headquarters' lobby. Every visitor seeing this sculpture must puzzle over the significance of something that doesn't highlight the most clever product of Merck, the most profitable product, or the most scientifically advanced offering of the company. Instead, it is a monument to human and corporate decency.

The second sculpture is at the Carter Center, a nongovernmental organization, where it serves as a symbol of hope in the midst of world problems. It is a statement that individuals, such as President Carter, can make a difference.

The third sculpture is in the lobby of the World Bank. This is perhaps the most unusual location for the statue, as it is in an institution that frequently asserts that it is not a health agency but a bank. Yet its visitors now see a reminder that the World Bank has mobilized the riches of the world to improve the health of the poorest of the poor.

The fourth and final copy is at the WHO in Geneva, an institution that originally failed to find a suitable mechanism to use the drug.

Jonas Salk said evolution will be what we want it to be, and that the only successful way to predict the future is to invent it. The Mectizan program is inventing the future, by not being tied to history:

- History would never have given a reason to believe that a pharmaceutical company would give a major amount of a drug free—forever!
- History could not have predicted a coalition that would be so broad, so committed, so productive.
- History would not have given us great confidence that communities would manage their own distribution program.
- History certainly would not have predicted results better than the most optimistic predictions.

On September 5, 2002, the 250 millionth treatment with Mectizan was celebrated, in Bombani village, Tanga region, Tanzania. It was a moment to praise things falling together rather than things falling apart. A moment to celebrate not only wisdom, which is knowing what to do next, but virtue, which is doing it. One speaker quoted William Penn, "To help mend the world is true religion."

By early 2021, Merck had donated 5 billion doses of Mectizan, for the annual treatment of entire populations in communities where the disease is transmitted. The Mectizan program is overseen by the Task Force for Global Health in Atlanta, Georgia (the Task Force for Child Survival's current name). After three decades of application, the incidence of the disease and blindness has been sharply reduced. Approximately 250 million treatments a year are being given. Surveillance and research programs monitor progress and suggest new approaches for total eradication.

Lymphatic Filariasis

Lymphatic filariasis is caused by a thread-like worm of the genus *Wuchereria*. It is spread by night-biting mosquitoes; the adult worm in humans lives in the lymphatic system. The worms block the flow of lymph, causing swelling of the legs (called elephantiasis) or scrotum. The disfigurement often leads to people being shunned, and the swelling makes it difficult to do farming or other work.

Fortunately, the philanthropy of Merck did not end with Mectizan and onchocerciasis. Next, it took on lymphatic filariasis. This is a story of serendipity.

It began at a Mectizan committee meeting in Clermont, France, on Thursday, October 17, 1996. Dr. Eric Ottesen, then working for WHO, gave a presentation on combining Mectizan and Albendazole for the treatment of lymphatic filariasis. Either drug alone was limited in value, he reported. However, when the two drugs were combined, the results were very encouraging.

Suddenly, the discussion became animated. The Mectizan program had shown what could happen when corporations became interested in neglected diseases. The committee had many members actively involved in that field, and any promising therapy was of consequence. Ottesen said Albendazole was produced by SmithKlein Beecham. However, no one at the meeting knew anyone high enough in that company to discuss a drug donation. The discussion continued at dinner and the next morning at breakfast.

At about 10 a.m. the next day, while chairing the meeting, I was called out of it to take a phone call from President Carter. He indicated that it was 5 a.m. in Atlanta, but he was so excited that he needed to talk. The night before, he had given a talk at Africare in Washington, DC. He subsequently had had dinner with Jan Leschly, who chaired Africare's board. Leschly talked about his admiration for the Merck gift of Mectizan and asked Carter for any suggestions he might have on how Leschly could benefit global health in a similar way.

I asked Carter what Leschly's position was, and Carter responded that he was the CEO of SmithKlein Beecham! I brought this news back to the Mectizan committee meeting. And by that afternoon, Carter had a tentative commitment for Albendazole to initiate a program against lymphatic filariasis!

It took several years to activate that program as neither company was willing to do field trials on the possible adverse effects of combining the two drugs. WHO initiated a meeting in Amsterdam to seek solutions to this problem. WHO asked me to chair the meeting. Early in the discussion, the participants concluded that the same dilemma had existed with vaccines. WHO had initiated studies on the use of simultaneous multiple antigens made by various companies. WHO could do the same for the use of these two drugs. The barrier was removed, studies were conducted, and a program was developed with drug gifts from both companies.

Even more good news followed when it was found, some years later, that the addition of a third drug, diethylcarbamazine (DEC), improved effectiveness. The Task Force for Global Health now coordinates a global program based on drug donations that permits annual administration of the three drugs (Mectizan, Albendazole, DEC) to entire villages. By early 2021, 16 countries had become free of the disease.

Helminths

As benefits accrued from the programs against river blindness and lymphatic filariasis, global health workers concerned with a host of other neglected diseases grew more confident. With the support of Glaxo-SmithKline, Johnson & Johnson, and the End Fund, the Task Force for Global Health became involved in finding ways to reduce the burden of soil-transmitted helminths.

Helminths are large multicellular worms. In their adult form, they do not multiply in humans; larval forms from outside the human body are required. The most common worms in the group are roundworms. These are treated effectively by Mectizan. And they are large enough that people see them being passed in their stools. The incidence of such helminths has been reduced in areas with river blindness programs. The other two problems in this group include hookworms (one of the earliest programs sponsored a century ago in the United States by the Rockefeller Foundation; see chapter 11) and whipworms.

The worms compete for nutrition with the infected person, and hookworms consume blood, often leading to anemia. All these worms have the capacity to hinder growth, causing stunting and reduced cognitive abilities. They are a significant and often hidden burden of living in poor areas of the world.

Programs to combat helminths combine direct treatment of populations, improved sanitation facilities, and education about hygiene practices. While some may not regard such programs as being as glamorous as surgery, they are an important approach to improving health, education, and energy levels of the populace.

Hepatitis

Hepatitis was a wastebasket of diseases 60 years ago. Now, we have good information on a variety of viruses that cause hepatitis, but we also understand that two viruses, hepatitis B and hepatitis C, often lead to cirrhosis of the liver or liver cancer. In many countries, hepatitis B is acquired early in life and eventually leads to the most common cancer in those countries. Over the years, aggressive research programs and field trials have led to vaccines for both hepatitis A and B, but also to effective treatment for hepatitis C. In my lifetime, our understanding of the disease has progressed from being a mystery to understanding its life cycle, creating vaccines, and having a treatment. The hepatitis B vaccine prevents an infectious disease that, in turn, causes a chronic disease; thus, we now have a vaccine to prevent a significant cancer.

Again, the corporate world has combined with the Task Force for Global Health to organize supplies and support to reduce global hepatitis B and C rates to low levels by 2030.

Trachoma

About 80 million people in the world have an eye infection called trachoma. It is an inflammation of the conjunctiva, especially on the inside of the eyelids. The result is a roughening on the undersurface of the eyelid. If untreated, repeated infections result in blindness. The disease is caused by *Chlamydia trachomatis* and is spread from person to person by secretions on towels or hands; it can even be transmitted by flies. Fortunately, the condition is treatable by topical or oral antibiotics.

The problem, of course, is that antibiotics have not been available in areas where the disease is common—or they are too expensive for the patients experiencing the disease. Again, a drug company, Pfizer, has come to the rescue to provide a drug, Azithromycin, which can be given to persons over six months of age, and even to pregnant women.

Pfizer has joined with the International Trachoma Initiative and the Task Force for Global Health to make Azithromycin available. To date, they have provided almost 1 billion treatments. Almost 100 million persons are now treated each year with that drug, and 10 countries have already eliminated the problem.

This latest chapter in global health is changing the outlook for millions. In addition to the programs mentioned, corporation-sponsored programs exist for leprosy, influenza, training programs in public health, improved polio vaccines, and the provision of medical equipment to areas of need. Such public–private programs will only increase in the future.

Concluding Thoughts

Pharmaceutical companies have the staffing and resources to bring programs to scale. They have distribution capabilities that make it easier to work in low-income countries. These companies' motivations involve both the altruistic desires of management as well as the benefits to staff, who like to identify with a company doing work to improve global health. The experience of the last 35 years has not supported the critics who predicted companies would use such programs to their own advantage. The involvement of major companies has been a key boon to global health.

This book has highlighted many changes in the efforts to improve global health. At the same time, the problems have also changed. Highway injuries, global pandemics, population profiles, and disease patterns continue to evolve. During medical training in the 1950s and 1960s, I never heard predictions on the future likelihood of obesity. While attention was being given to tropical diseases, few were talking about hypertension and diabetes in poor countries. Suddenly, the chronic diseases are exploding faster than medical programs can respond. Pharmaceutical companies now have opportunities to expand their philanthropy into providing far more medications, at low cost, for poor countries.

Adulterated and mislabeled drugs are a constant problem in low-resource countries. Several years ago, two students from Ghana suggested a solution: companies could label each container with a code. The buyer could take a picture of the code, call a number, and verify that it was made by that company in the indicated dosage on the vial. Innovative opportunities abound.

CHAPTER 14

Pharmaceuticals and Other Global Health Topics

PAUL ELISH AND ALISON T. HOOVER

A consistent theme in medicine across history is the search for cures to the most recalcitrant diseases. That search—manifested in everything from herbalism to modern bench science—has given rise to the wealth of pharmaceuticals we know today. But when a miracle drug is discovered, the journey to widespread access and adoption has just begun. Armed conflict, inequity, antibiotic resistance, and many other factors can jeopardize even the most remarkable pharmaceutical advances. The following chapter explores the multifaceted, inspiring, and fraught story of pharmaceuticals in global health.

The History of Quinine

More than 400 years ago, cinchona bark emerged as a treatment for malarial fevers in the Andes Mountains. The exact details of the discovery remain a mystery. Legends talk of pumas seen drinking cinchona-infused water to cure their shivering, or an earthquake that felled cinchona trees into a lake and made the lake's water medicinal. One of the most common stories about cinchona bark's origins recounts how healers used the bark to save the Viceroy of Peru's wife, the Countess of Chinchón, from malaria, though it was actually the viceroy himself who was cured using cinchona bark powder in May 1631.[1]

While there are no direct accounts of the bark's discovery, it is clear that it was originally discovered by Indigenous healers. Several writings from Spanish physicians in the mid-17th century explain that Jesuit missionaries in present-day Peru and Ecuador observed Indigenous people drinking water infused with pulverized cinchona to cure chills. One such account comes from Diego Salado Garzés, who authored a medical treatise at the University of Seville in the 1670s. Salado Garzés wrote that the Jesuits began using cinchona bark to treat malarial fevers "after observing that the Indians took it when shivering from cold after swimming in iced water or from coldness of the snow and stopped trembling within a short time."[1]

Today, hundreds of years after its discovery in Ecuador's tropical forests, the bark's active compound—quinine—remains on the World Health Organization's list of essential medicines.[2] Over the centuries, this wonder drug spread across the Atlantic, played a role in the United States's westward expansion, and was of critical military importance in the Pacific during World War II.[2,3] Quinine's history set many early precedents for modern global health. It demonstrates the power of Indigenous medicine, the interconnectedness of ecology and health, the impact of government economic policy on pharmaceuticals, and stark inequality in pharmaceutical access.

Quinine's Roots in Herbalism

Like many pharmaceuticals, quinine has its roots in tropical forests. *Cinchona* is a genus of flowering plants in the *Rubiaceae* family (the same botanical family as coffee), which is native to the rainforests in the central and northern Andes Mountains. These rainforests on mountainous terrain, or "cloud forests," are biodiversity hotspots.[4] The use of cinchona bark for malaria is thought to have originated in the cloud forests around present-day Loja, Ecuador. This region of southern Ecuador has an especially high degree of biodiversity because of the concentration of ecosystems, ranging from cloud forest to deciduous forest to desert, within a relatively small area.[5] Quinine's origins are thus an example of how biodiverse tropical rainforests can function as nature's medicine cabinet.

Early European descriptions of cinchona bark gave credit to "Indians" for discovering its medicinal properties. Accounts describe how cinchona bark was dried, ground into a powder, and mixed into liquids like water or wine to be drunk. The Jesuits were the first to bring cinchona bark to Europe, when they introduced it as "Jesuit's powder" in Rome in the 1640s. As with many modern pharmaceuticals, the drug's availability was initially limited to elites. In England, London's high society began experimenting with cinchona in the 1650s; the poor in southeastern England who suffered recurring malaria epidemics had no such access. The Jesuits also used cinchona bark to successfully treat China's Qing emperor in 1693.[3] But the skepticism and conspiracies that shrouded cinchona bark represent another parallel with modern pharmaceuticals. Some historians believe Oliver Cromwell died of malaria, and if this is true, that he died in part because he refused to take a medicine associated with Catholic Jesuits.[6] In the American Revolution, both the British and colonial rebels used "Peruvian bark" to treat malaria, but many remained skeptical of its effectiveness since drug grinders frequently mixed it with other ingredients.[3]

Early accounts of quinine illustrate an important nuance in colonial attitudes about medical knowledge. Europeans considered colonized peoples' medical practices to be quackery or, in some cases, satanic. However, European attitudes about Indigenous herbal knowledge were significantly more positive. Dutch physicians in colonial Asia frequently expressed admiration for local people's knowledge of herbs.[7] The Portuguese were similarly enthusiastic about foreign herbal remedies; the famed 16th-century Portuguese Jewish physician and herbalist Garcia d'Orta wrote the *Colloquies on the Simples, Drugs, and Materia Medica of India*, which collected Indigenous herbal knowledge from Goa, India, and its surroundings. Europe was also quick to import herbal remedies in the age of exploration. One of the earliest examples was the attempted use of guaiac from Hispaniola and "China root" from Goa to fight Europe's syphilis outbreaks in the early 1500s.[7]

And the Spanish, despite their infamous Inquisition, accepted Indigenous herbalism. When Spanish royal physician Francisco Hernández led a botanical expedition in Mexico in the 1570s, he wrote:

> I marveled, in this and in innumerable other herbs, which are nameless among us, how in the Indies, where people are so uncultured and barbaric, there are so many herbs, some with known uses and some without, but there is almost none, which is not known to them and given a particular name.[8]

Even though the Spanish viewed other Andean healers as idolatrous, they recognized the impressive knowledge of herbalists in the Andes. The Inca, themselves, held herbalism in high esteem. The 16th-century mestizo chronicler Inca Garcilaso de la Vega wrote how the Inca Empire's greatest herbalists personally provided care to the Inca kings and their families in the pre-Columbian era. Shared respect for herbalism across Andean Indigenous peoples and Spanish colonizers was also helped by some similarities between the European humoral understanding of medicine and the Andean medical understanding, which similarly focused on balance between such things as hot and cold temperatures.[5]

The Road to Mass Production

Cinchona bark and quinine's history becomes more recognizable to modern eyes when scientific laboratories began investigating the bark in the 19th century. In 1820, French scientists Pierre-Joseph Pelletier and his student Joseph Bienaimé Caventou isolated quinine and cinchonine from the bark as part of the broader emergence of modern alkaloidal chemistry. In the 1830s and 1840s, Europeans and North Americans began using isolated quinine in lieu of bark.[3]

After quinine was isolated, there was an international race to capture the quinine market. This included a push to modernize cinchona bark's supply chain. The early supply chain involved incredible toil. Indigenous people in the Andes would find the trees in the forest, strip off their bark, load it on mules, and either bring it to Spanish ports or float it as contraband to Portuguese or Dutch merchants on the Amazon River. This approach began to fade when, in the 1850s, the Dutch and British sent botanists to collect cinchona seedlings and established cinchona plantations outside of South America. British attempts in India and modern-day Sri Lanka in the 1860s were modestly successful, but the Dutch ultimately dominated the market. They focused heavily on cultivating high-quinine specimens in their plantations in modern-day Indonesia. They grafted the highest yield sapling stalks onto the roots of other trees to make "super trees." By the early 20th century, 90% of the world's quinine supply came from the Dutch-held island of Java in modern Indonesia.[3]

In a precursor to the modern international pharmaceutical industry, global economic policy dramatically shaped access to quinine. The biggest market for quinine in the mid-19th century was among settlers in the United States west of the Appalachian Mountains, but consistent quinine treatment remained expensive and out of reach for poor farmers. This changed when the US Congress abolished duties on imported quinine in 1879. Dutch and British producers flooded the quinine market, and prices in the United States plummeted. Rural Americans began to take more regular and larger doses of quinine, contributing to malaria's decline in North America. In contrast, colonial administrations did not usually fund quinine for Indigenous people. Indigenous malaria patients generally could not afford quinine and did not have access to it unless it was distributed by medical missionaries.[3] A medication that was discovered by Indigenous herbalists was not widely available to Indigenous populations under colonial rule.

Quinine's importance reached another crest during World War II, when Japanese forces captured the Dutch colonies in modern Indonesia and cut off almost all of the Allies' quinine supply, in 1942. The supply cut initiated yet another race in the antimalarial pharmaceutical sector, this time for a synthetic alternative. More than 14,000 compounds were tested against malaria in a US Government–funded program that would be used as a model for the US National Institutes of Health after the war. Two synthetic antimalaria drugs, Atabrine and chloroquine, were identified in 1943 and 1945, respectively.[3] Quinine's longstanding role as the only available antimalarial drug came to an end.

Despite the discovery of synthetic alternatives to quinine, traditional and Indigenous medicine's role in the fight against malaria wasn't over. As synthetic antimalarials became more popular, the threat of drug-resistant malaria grew stronger due to overuse. This was especially true in the Vietnam War, when both the US and Vietnamese forces used chloroquine extensively.[9,10] North Vietnamese forces pleaded with China for new antimalarial drugs. In response, Mao Tse-tung ordered the creation of a top-secret state mission called Project 523 on May 23, 1967, with two research groups: one investigated synthetic antimalarial drug development and the other examined traditional Chinese medicines for potential antimalarial compounds.[11]

The second group enlisted traditional Chinese medicine doctors to travel around China and collect folk remedies as part of the "barefoot doctors" scheme. The group tested different traditional remedies until arriving at *Artemisia annua* (called *Ging Hao* in Chinese and "sweet wormword" in English). The first mention of Ging Hao is in the *Fifty-Two Remedies*, a medical treatise written on silk and found in a tomb dating to 168 BCE.[11,12] Hundreds of years later, the first recorded mention of Ging Hao's antimalarial properties was written in 340 CE by Ge Hong, an alchemist and medical expert in China's Eastern Jin dynasty. By extracting artemisinin from Ging Hao in the early 1970s and developing more artemisinin derivatives between 1976 and 1978, the Project 523 team translated ancient herbal knowledge into the most powerful pharmaceuticals that we have today for severe malaria.[11]

Through the story of quinine, we see how ecology, government economic policy, and inequality can all shape health outcomes related to pharmaceuticals. The stories of quinine and artemisinin are also examples of the power of traditional herbalism. They demonstrate that medicinal and herbal knowledge can transcend cultures, medical paradigms, and centuries to save lives around the globe.

Tuberculosis and the Threat of Multidrug Resistance

In the story of quinine and artemisinin, we see how certain pharmaceutical discoveries can have staying power across centuries. The string of antibiotic discoveries from the 1800s onward can also give the impression of linear progress over infectious disease. The reality is that many of humanity's antibiotic victories are in jeopardy. The US Centers for Disease Control and Prevention's 2019 Antibiotic Resistance Threats Report estimated that in the United States alone, more than 2.8 million antibiotic-resistant infections occur annually, leading to more than 35,000 deaths.[13] Worldwide annual antibiotic-resistant fatalities are estimated at 700,000 but are projected to reach 10 million by 2050 if stronger policies against drug resistance are not instituted.[14]

The driving force of antibiotic resistance is overuse and misuse of antibiotic medications, which places pressure on bacteria and fungi populations to develop antibiotic-resistant genes. Overuse and misuse of antibiotics take a variety of forms. Antibiotics are frequently over-prescribed by healthcare providers, and patients' inadequate adherence to antibiotic regimens can stoke resistance further.[15,16] Outside of healthcare settings, antibiotics are used heavily in livestock to promote growth and prevent disease—about 80% of antibiotics sold in the United States are administered to farm animals. These antibiotics are then consumed by humans when they eat meat. Agricultural antibiotics also enter the broader water supply when excreted in livestock's urine and feces or when sprayed directly into the environment, as seen with tetracyclines and streptomycin sprayed on fruit trees to combat plant disease.[15]

The history of tuberculosis (TB) is one example of how the world's most pivotal antibiotic advances are at risk. In high-income settings, TB can seem like a cultural artifact. TB ravaged Europe and North

America in the 19th century but was famously romanticized by artists. In high society, pulmonary tuberculosis, known popularly as "consumption" because it appeared to consume sufferers, had a favorable association with fragility and attractiveness. Women's fashion promoted thinness, a pale complexion, and red cheeks in imitation of those sick with tuberculosis.[17] The idea of an artistic death at the hands of tuberculosis lived on in pop culture in the 21st century, as seen in films like *Moulin Rouge!*

The reality is that the global burden of tuberculosis remains both unromantic and enormous. About a quarter of all people are infected with TB, and 5% to 10% of those infected will fall ill with active TB disease during their lifetime. In 2021, 1.6 million people died of TB, making it the second-leading cause of death from a single infectious agent. An estimated 500,000 people worldwide are infected annually with multidrug-resistant (MDR) TB, defined as tuberculosis that is resistant to the first-line anti-TB drugs isoniazid and rifampin. There are ominous signs that inadequate treatment of MDR TB is fueling additional cases that are resistant to most, and perhaps all, antituberculosis drugs.[18]

The present-day burden of TB follows on thousands of years of TB mortality. Spinal TB has been identified in bones dating to 8000 BCE, as well as human remains from Ancient Egypt and pre-Columbian civilizations in the Americas. Literature in India dating to 1500 BCE also comments on the existence of TB. In Ancient Greece, Hippocrates (460–370 BCE) wrote that tuberculosis was one of the most common diseases in the period, and he warned against trying to treat patients with advanced TB since they would inevitably die and tarnish physicians' reputations. There were relatively few advances in understanding TB until the 19th century. Although scientists in Europe in the 1500s and 1600s gained a better idea of the anatomical effects of TB through autopsies, the mechanism of infection remained a mystery.[19] In the 19th century, tuberculosis accounted for about a quarter of all deaths in Massachusetts and New York and killed about one-quarter of Europe's population.[18]

After thousands of years of tuberculosis deaths, discoveries in the late 1800s substantially enhanced human understanding of the disease. On March 24, 1882, Robert Koch gave a landmark lecture, "The Etiology of Tuberculosis," at a meeting of the Physiological Society at Berlin's Charité Hospital.[19] Koch produced evidence of the bacteria causing tuberculosis. Special staining techniques under the microscope allowed him to visualize the slender rods of *Mycobacterium tuberculosis*. When he developed cultures of the bacteria and injected them into laboratory animals, the animals developed TB.[18]

In the following decade, the fight against TB gained another important tool. Wilhelm Conrad Röntgen discovered X-rays in 1895, which allowed physicians to diagnose and monitor the course and severity of TB in patients.[19] In the 1930s, lung collapse therapy also became a common, effective TB treatment, and the bacillus Calmette–Guérin (BCG) vaccine was first used in 1921; BCG continues to be used in higher-risk settings and high-risk patients against the most dangerous forms of non-pulmonary TB.[19]

The big breakthrough in TB treatment came during World War II. Selman Waksman, a scientist at Rutgers University, contributed decades of research on soil fungi and bacteria that could stop bacterial growth.[18,19] In 1940, Waksman's scientific team experimented with a soil fungus and isolated actinomycin, a highly toxic antibiotic. Although actinomycin was too toxic for clinical treatment, the finding soon led to the discovery of another antibiotic, streptomycin, which was appropriate for clinical use, in 1943. In November 1944, a severely ill TB patient at the Mayo Clinic in Rochester, Minnesota, was successfully treated with streptomycin. The 21-year-old woman recovered and went on to have three healthy children.[19]

New antibiotics contributed to profound reductions in tuberculosis mortality, but early on, there were warning signs. Within months of streptomycin's introduction, mutant strains of TB began to appear that were resistant to the antibiotic. In the world's first modern randomized, controlled trial, in 1948, the British Medical Research Council investigated streptomycin's effectiveness and found that many patients were cured, but a substantial number of patients relapsed with cases that were resistant to that antibiotic.[18] Fortunately, an expanding arsenal of drugs helped combat resistance. P-aminosalicylic acid, isoniazid, pyrazinamide, cycloserine, ethambutol, and rifampin all entered into use by the early 1960s. Aminoglycosides and more recently developed quinolones (discovered, coincidentally, during the synthesis of antimalarial quinine compounds[20]) are reserved for drug-resistant cases, and certain drugs (namely, isoniazid, rifampin, and ethambutol) are especially effective for preventing resistance.[19] Today, multidrug treatment regimens are recommended to prevent resistance.[18]

Funding patterns contributed to TB remaining a persistent issue and to the rise of MDR TB. In the past century, tuberculosis became a disease of low- and middle-income countries. Its spread is facilitated by poverty; people who are malnourished and living in crowded conditions are especially susceptible. Yet once TB was more properly controlled in the United States after antibiotic discoveries, the US Government's funding for TB drug, diagnostic, and vaccine research was dramatically cut.[18] International health donors and policymakers began to favor more targeted and inexpensive primary care interventions in the 1980s. Tuberculosis treatment, with its lengthy follow-up periods, did not appear cost-effective to donors, who hoped to find less expensive solutions by investing in research and development. Even as funders shied away from TB, it remained the leading killer of young adults globally in the 20th century.[18]

Funding for tuberculosis treatment regained some momentum in 1993 when the World Bank began using disability-adjusted life years (DALYs) when choosing health interventions to support. DALYs helped estimate interventions' cost-effectiveness by calculating the number of additional healthy years of life that interventions could deliver in target populations. Suddenly, when accounting for DALYs, short-term antituberculosis medication regimes appeared highly cost-effective. WHO responded with robust support for the directly observed therapy, short-course (DOTS) strategy, in which tuberculosis programs would follow a simple, algorithmic process. TB would be diagnosed through smear microscopy, and treatment would only use first-line antituberculosis medications.[18]

The increased funding for DOTS did save lives, but it came at the price of increased drug resistance. Smear microscopy has low sensitivity and has no ability to detect drug-resistant *M. tuberculosis*, and first-line medications alone do not adequately address resistance. The DOTS approach left the door open to resistant TB strains just as the HIV epidemic contributed to further TB outbreaks by compromising patients' immune systems.[18]

By the mid-1990s, MDR TB had spread globally. In some high-income settings, the response adequately addressed drug resistance. In the United States in the late 1980s and early 1990s, public health officials responded to MDR TB outbreaks through a national plan aimed specifically at fighting and researching drug-resistant TB. New York City's TB program used mycobacterial culture for more accurate diagnosis, drug-susceptibility testing, and second-line medications to fight resistant strains.[18]

Unlike New York City's strategy, WHO continued promoting the combination of smear microscopy diagnosis and first-line medications. This strategy did have impressive results in countries like Peru, where the DOTS strategy made tuberculosis medication therapy widely available. But TB outbreaks in northern shanty towns in Lima, Peru, included many drug-resistant cases.[18] Jim Kim and Paul Farmer of Partners In Health were intent on intervening to apply the MDR TB standard of care applied in the United States. WHO opposed the plan, but Partners In Health secured funding from the Bill & Melinda Gates Foundation to show the approach could work in the poorest of environments. WHO had encouraged Peru to opt for the lower-cost approach but ended up so impressed by the results that it offered Kim a position (Bill Foege, pers. comm., 2023).

While some progress has been made globally, MDR TB remains a daunting problem. In 2017, it was estimated that just 25% of more than 500,000 people with MDR-TB worldwide were diagnosed and on treatment. Only about 55% of MDR TB patients on treatment complete the treatment regimen successfully.[21] But a historic milestone was reached in 2022: WHO approved a new six-month drug regimen composed of bedaquiline, pretomanid, linezolid, and moxifloxacin (BPaLM) for patients with multidrug- or rifampicin-resistant (MDR/RR) TB.[22] The BPaLM regimen could usher in better outcomes, shorter treatment, and better quality of life for those living with drug-resistant TB.[23]

TB is not the only disease with issues of drug resistance. CDC's 2019 Antibiotic Resistance Threats Report identified 5 bacteria and fungi as "urgent threats" and 11 as "serious threats." The diseases caused by these threats vary. The urgent threats—those that are considered to pose the greatest danger—include Carbapenem-resistant *Acinetobacter* (causing pneumonia and wound, bloodstream, and urinary tract infections), *Clostridiodes difficiles* (causing life-threatening diarrhea and colon inflammation), Carbapenem-resistant Enterobacterales, and drug-resistant gonorrhea (which increases the risk of getting and giving HIV and causes ectopic pregnancy and infertility).[24]

All of these antibiotic-resistant diseases require global solutions that effectively tackle antibiotic overuse and address drug-resistant outbreaks. The history of TB serves as an important cautionary tale for what can happen in the absence of strong international commitments to global solutions. TB appeared antiquated in high-income countries, and over several decades there was correspondingly lukewarm support for TB research and comprehensive MDR TB interventions in low- and middle-income countries. This pattern now threatens to convert TB from a disease of the past into a disease of the future.

Anthrax and Global Security

Another catalyst for pharmaceutical development has stemmed from an unlikely place: national defense and anti-bioterrorism efforts.

On October 2, 2001, just three weeks after the September 11 terrorist attacks, Robert "Bob" Stevens stumbled into a Florida emergency room, delirious with fever.[25] An infectious disease consultant was called, and the doctor was surprised to see the classic, large, boxcar-shaped *Bacillus anthracis* (the bacteria that causes anthrax infection) under the microscope. Two days later, Stevens was diagnosed with the first case of inhalation anthrax in the United States since 1976.[26] Only 18 known cases of inhalation anthrax had occurred in the country before Stevens, and all were the result of workplace exposure to naturally occurring anthrax, usually through animal products. But Stevens, a newspaper photo editor, had no risk of workplace exposure. As it would turn out, he would be the first of many Americans to have been exposed to anthrax through an intentional act of bioterrorism.

Over the next seven weeks, public panic ensued as letters mailed to news agencies along the East Coast and to two senators' offices were discovered to have been coated with a white powder containing anthrax spores. As many as 10,000 people were considered at risk of possible exposure to anthrax and were treated with antibiotics as a post-exposure prophylaxis.[25] Billions of dollars were spent on cleaning contaminated facilities, testing exposed individuals, and conducting a federal investigation. Ultimately 22 cases of anthrax were diagnosed, including in both the recipients of the letters and the postal workers who handled them. Five people died of their exposure, including Stevens.

The FBI, CDC, and state and local authorities launched "Amerithrax," an unprecedented dual criminal and epidemiologic investigation to determine the source of the letters. Dr. Steven Hatfill was initially identified as the principal person of interest, given his position as a scientist at the US Army's Medical Research Institute of Infectious Diseases (USAMRIID), where US stocks of anthrax spores were stored. He was one of the few people who had access to the substance. He was eventually cleared of wrongdoing and successfully sued the US Justice Department for defamation, winning a $5.8 million settlement.

The final investigative summary was not published until February 2010, eight years later. It concluded that Bruce Ivins, another research scientist at USAMRIID, acted alone in planning and implementing the anthrax letters. The investigative summary cited, as the definitive proof, a genetic link between the anthrax spores in the letters and spores that Ivins had developed and maintained under his role as a microbiologist studying vaccines and cures for anthrax exposure at USAMRIID. But Ivins was not charged; after becoming a person of interest, being put under constant surveillance, and being banned from his lab, he developed severe depression and took his own life in 2008.

Alongside the inability to prosecute Ivins, the conclusions of the Amerithrax investigation remain somewhat in question. At the FBI's request, a separate panel of experts gathered by the National Academy of Sciences conducted an independent evaluation of the genetic analysis of the anthrax spores in February 2011; the panel deemed the scientific evidence put forth in the Amerithrax investigative summary insufficient to definitively prove Ivins was the culprit.[25] The genetic testing techniques used to trace the anthrax strain back to Ivins' lab were novel. The panel determined that, while the microbial forensics were consistent with Ivins' strain, guilt could not be definitively determined. To date, there is still no conclusive answer on who was responsible for the 2001 anthrax attack, nor are there scientific techniques that could definitively determine guilt.

A Brief History of Anthrax

Though its use as a bioweapon has been reserved to the last century, the bacterium that causes an anthrax infection, *B. anthracis*, is ancient. It is believed to have originated in Egypt and Mesopotamia, and references to the bacteria date back to around 700 BC. Anthrax is believed to have caused the fifth of Egypt's 10 plagues and is likely what Homer referred to in the *Iliad*, when he described a "burning wind of plague" that affected "pack animals first, and dogs, but soldiers too." The bacteria are naturally occurring; animal herbivores are the natural host. Humans commonly acquire an infection through contact with infected animals or animal products. The link between anthrax infections and the animal hair industry was so common in the 1800s that anthrax was referred to as the "wool sorter's disease." *B. anthracis* is a particularly sturdy bacterium, able to transform into spores that can survive in soil for decades. Early disease control interventions, which entailed culling large populations of livestock and burying their carcasses, sowed potential epidemics, the bacteria lying in wait for a single till of the soil.

Anthrax infections can take three forms, depending upon how they are acquired: cutaneous, commonly acquired through butchering, skinning, or handling infected hides; gastrointestinal, through consuming contaminated meat; or inhalation, through breathing in spores in the air. For the anthrax attack of 2001, 11 case-patients had cutaneous exposure from touching the powder, and the other 11 had inhalational exposure through breathing in the spores released during the opening of the letter. Inhalation anthrax is the most fatal form of infection; cutaneous is the most common.[26]

Germ Theory and Koch versus Pasteur

Anthrax is more than a villain in history, however. The study of anthrax led to the discovery of germ theory and the development of Koch's postulates, the four criteria used to determine a causal link between a germ and a disease. (For more on the germ theory, see chapter 3.) Robert Koch was born in northwest Germany in 1843.[27] He was a physician with a keen curiosity for natural science, which led his wife to give him a microscope that would ultimately change the way society understood disease.

After being appointed district medical officer, Koch sought to understand the anthrax epidemic that was ravaging both livestock and humans in his community. At the time, it was understood that rod-shaped structures were present in the blood of infected animals and that injecting the blood of an infected animal into another animal would transmit the disease. Some pastures were known to be dangerous for livestock grazing, but little else was known or understood about anthrax.

Koch designed elaborate animal studies that led to the development of artificial culturing techniques. He cultured (or grew) B. anthracis in warm, moist, and aerated environments and observed its transformation into spores. This explained how the bacteria could survive for so long in soil, despite blood losing its ability to transmit disease just a few days after a host was infected. Koch then wisely recommended alternative practices for disposing of the remains of infected animals in his community to preclude spores from forming in soil.

Koch announced in 1876 that his studies proved causality—that indeed the germ *B. anthracis* caused an anthrax infection. Germ theory preceded Koch, but at the time of his experiments it was controversial and had little societal acceptance. But Koch's carefully designed experiments became the most conclusive evidence of germ theory to date and earned him renown in the microbiology community.[28]

One person was not particularly thrilled with Koch's advancements: Louis Pasteur. Koch, a German, and Pasteur, a Frenchman, became scientists during the Franco-German War of 1870–1871. Their nations' feud quickly resonated in their personal and professional relationship, as Koch rose in the microbiology community. Pasteur had been the leading microbiologist of the day, advocating for broader acceptance of germ theory. But when Koch and his findings were taken more seriously and more readily accepted, from a newcomer and a German no less, Pasteur was livid.

Pasteur argued that Koch's studies and findings were insufficient to determine causality and remained inferences. Fueled by his new rivalry, Pasteur set about to definitively prove causality through the development of an anthrax vaccine. In a now infamous experiment, before a large audience, he inoculated 31 livestock animals (a mix of sheep, goats, and cows) in a village outside of Paris, Pouilly-le-Fort, in 1881, with a vaccine using attenuated live organisms.[29] Thirty days later, the inoculated 31 animals and 29 non-inoculated ones were injected with a virulent anthrax culture. All 24 unvaccinated sheep and the 1 unvaccinated goat died from the infection; the 4 unvaccinated cows lived but became very ill. All 31 vaccinated animals survived. Pasteur claimed this was the definitive proof Europe had been seeking of causality and that he, in fact, had now proven germ theory.

Koch was enraged that Pasteur had used his research in the vaccine development process and not credited him appropriately. A series of public critiques ensued, with barbs tossed from both sides. Koch accused Pasteur of sloppy study design and implementation, and inconclusive or irrelevant results. Pasteur was a chemist, not a physician, leading Koch to lob additional insults onto his contemporary: "Pasteur is not a physician, and one cannot expect him to make sound judgments about pathological processes and the symptoms of disease."[30]

But Pasteur did produce a successful vaccine. His anthrax vaccine for livestock was the first effective bacterial vaccine and the second vaccine ever produced, after the smallpox vaccine. Anthrax vaccines built off his foundational research continue to be used in livestock around the world today. Routine animal vaccinations, combined with improvements in animal-processing practices, have led to major declines in the number of anthrax cases in humans.[26]

Bioterrorism

Just when naturally occurring cases of anthrax were on the decline, anthrax as a bioweapon hit the scene. The year 2001 was the first time anthrax was used as a weapon of bioterrorism in the general public, but its first use as a bioweapon took place during World War I. It is likely that the German army infected livestock and animal feed that was traded to the Allied Nations by neutral partners, leading to the death of 200 Argentinian mules in 1917 and 1918.[26]

The use of anthrax and other biological and chemical forms of warfare during World War I led to the creation, in 1925, of the Geneva Protocol for the Prevention of the Use in War of Asphyxiating, Poisonous or other Gases, and of Bacteriological Methods of Warfare. The treaty had a loophole: it did not outlaw research on or production of biological agents—it only outlawed their use. In 1932, Japan began producing anthrax and conducted experiments on prisoners in Japanese-occupied Manchuria. During this time, Japan is believed to have sprayed anthrax and other biological agents on homes in at least 11 cities.

Great Britain conducted a large-scale bioweapon experiment on a small island off the coast of Scotland during World War II. Gruinard Island was requisitioned by the government, filled with sheep, and doused in anthrax through the detonation of bombs across the island. All the sheep died from their exposure, but the most significant finding from this experiment was how long anthrax lingered in the environment after its release. The island was considered uninhabitable after decontamination efforts failed in the face of the sturdy bacteria. It wasn't until 1986 that decontamination efforts were renewed—a process that entailed removing the top layer of soil and drenching the island with a concentration of formaldehyde diluted with seawater. The island was officially deemed habitable in 1990, a full 48 years later, after a flock of sheep remained healthy on the island.

The United States started its own bioweapons program during World War II, in 1942, with testing sites in Mississippi and Utah. More than 5,000 bombs were equipped with anthrax to be used in retaliation for any German attacks. The program was expanded during the Korean War and included a component focused on vaccines and treatment for soldiers exposed to anthrax in the line of duty. The United States—and other nations—had amassed an extensive supply of bioweapons by the 1960s, causing international concern. A conversation begun by Great Britain and furthered by the Warsaw Pact nations led to President Richard Nixon's terminating the US bioweapons program via executive order in 1969. That order stipulated the end of research and production in tandem with destruction of all stockpiled bioweapons. The only elements of the bioweapon program that were preserved were efforts to develop vaccines, treatments, and diagnostic tests. The rest of the world soon followed. In 1972, over 100 countries, including the Soviet Union, ratified the Convention on the Prohibition of the Development, Production and Stockpiling of Bacteriological (Biological) and Toxin Weapons and on their Destruction.

Given that the Soviet Union had ratified the treaty, it raised eyebrows when reports of an anthrax outbreak surfaced in Sverdlovsk, Russia, in 1980. Though it was heavily denied at the time, it eventually came to light years later that improperly installed air filters at a Soviet military microbiology facility with ongoing anthrax biological weapon testing was to blame for at least 66 human deaths.

As with the controversy around Pasteur's livestock vaccine, developing a vaccine for humans faced its own challenges. The Soviet Union was the first to develop an anthrax vaccine for humans, in the 1930s. The UK followed suit with its own vaccine in 1954, and the United States licensed its BioThrax vaccine in 1970.[31] In 1997, the Clinton administration implemented the Anthrax Vaccine Immunization Program, which mandated that active US military personnel receive Bio-Thrax vaccines. The mandate was unpopular, with numerous refusals on the basis of unknown long-term safety and efficacy, leading to court martials and rank demotions.[32] A legal injunction temporarily halted the program in 2004, but it was reinstated in 2006 after an FDA investigation confirmed its safety and efficacy.[33] The vaccinations are still required for any military members working in bioterrorism defense or deployed to Iraq, Afghanistan, or South Korea.

The threat and use of anthrax as a bioweapon sparked significant national security and public health reform. Bio-watch air-monitoring stations were installed, smallpox vaccines were stockpiled, and the Project BioShield Act was passed in 2004. The act resulted in billions of dollars of investment into research and development of next-generation therapies for bioweapon exposure. Protecting citizen health became a matter of national security, and funding flowed easily—at least, for a few years.[34] The United States has not experienced a bioterror event since 2001,* and attention has shifted to health security and preparedness.

Funding plays a central role in pharmaceuticals and global health. In addition to disaster preparedness and response, funding makes it possible to develop new drugs, respond to resistance, and keep medications affordable. But as with anthrax, funding comes and goes, and so does the affordability of medications.

---

* Though a confirmed instance of bioterror has not occurred, hoaxes continue. In 2020, Anthony Fauci, director of the National Institute of Allergy and Infectious Diseases, opened a letter containing a "puff of powder" that covered his face and chest. The substance turned out to be benign.[35]

Role of TRIPS Agreement in Global Pharmaceutical Access

Trade-related policies are the reason that the same medication can cost $1,000 in the United States, $10 in India, and be entirely unavailable for purchase in China. Global tugs-of-war over protection policies can yield drastically different access and costs for the same medication.

Taking a new drug to market is a lengthy, costly process, and the road to success is paved with failed attempts. Ninety percent of clinical drug development fails to get regulatory approval.[36] Of the 10% that succeeded in the United States in 2022, it took on average $2 billion and 14 years of development to bring a drug to the market.[37] The enormous investment that drug companies make in new drug development is motivated by the colossal profits possible from a successful drug. One US Government Accountability Office study found that the top 25 drug companies have an annual profit margin of 15–20%, compared to the largest 500 nondrug companies, which have an annual profit margin between 4% and 9%.[38]

The goal of intellectual property (IP) protection provisions is to ensure robust return on investment for companies that do succeed in bringing a novel drug to market. Most IP protections limit generic manufacturers from making and selling the drug more cheaply, at least for a period of time, to allow developers to transfer some of their costs to end users. But IP protections can also have significant negative public health consequences by inflating the cost of drugs, making them unaffordable to many who need them.

The IP policy tug-of-war has played out in the Trade-Related Aspects of Intellectual Property Rights (or TRIPS) Agreement, implemented by the World Trade Organization (WTO) in 1995. Under TRIPS, members of the WTO are required to make patents available for technological inventions to protect public health and improve equitable medication access.[39] It also stipulates uniform IP regulations across countries.[40] The negotiations that led to the TRIPS Agreement did not focus on public health, but they had major public health implications, especially for pharmaceutical access. The agreement required WTO members to institute 20-year patents for all technological fields, including pharmaceuticals. Before TRIPS, many countries did not assign patents for pharmaceuticals. TRIPS has manifested in highly varied access—and price tags—for the same medications in different countries.

Impact on Access to HIV Medication

It soon became clear that the TRIPS reforms would pose problems for people living with HIV, particularly in low- and middle-income countries (LMICs). Antiretroviral drugs and their groundbreaking ability to manage HIV infection as a chronic disease rather than a death sentence were introduced to the world in 1996, but they were not affordable for developing countries. One solution was for LMICs to produce generic equivalents domestically. Thailand and Brazil pursued this route, but TRIPS requirements limited their options. Brazil initially produced low-cost generics, but its government came under pressure from high-income countries to begin granting pharmaceutical patents, which it began doing in 1996. The price of antiretrovirals in Brazil quickly ballooned.[41]

India delayed implementation of its TRIPS-adherent Indian Patents Act until 2005. As a result, the country was able to dramatically expand antiretrovirals available to LMICs. Generic pharmaceutical companies in India faced fierce domestic competition, which kept prices low. The lack of pharmaceutical patents also allowed Indian companies to produce "fixed-dose combinations" that combined two or more medicines into one pill, further reducing prices. Whereas a triple-combination antiretroviral produced by the Indian company Cipla in 2001 cost $350 per year, the previous lowest price for the same drug combination from original manufacturers was about $1,000 per year.[41] Cipla was lauded for exposing the other manufacturers' abuse of their market monopoly while demonstrating the value of generic manufacturers in improving drug affordability.

South Africa, with the world's largest population of people living with HIV, amended its Medicines Act in 1997 to make antiretrovirals affordable and available to South African people living with HIV. In response, the South African government was met with a lawsuit in

1998 from 41 pharmaceutical companies that declared the amend-ments unlawful and noncompliant with the TRIPS Agreement.[41]

The lawsuit galvanized nongovernmental organizations and AIDS activists, who put forward compulsory licensing as a potential solu-tion. With a compulsory license, an entity other than the patent holder receives a license from a government to produce a patented product. The TRIPS Agreement allowed for compulsory licensing, though the interpretation and implementation varied. At the 2000 International AIDS Conference in Durban, South Africa, advocates organized a Global March for Treatment that demanded broad, equitable access to antiretrovirals.[41]

The advocacy paid off. In May 2000, five pharmaceutical companies unveiled price discounts on antiretrovirals and HIV diagnostics, but the prices were still higher than generics. Further global advocacy and public outcry led the 41 litigating drug companies to drop the case in South Africa. The advocacy also paved the way for the November 2001 Doha Declaration on the TRIPS Agreement and Public Health.[41] The Doha Declaration stated that the TRIPS Agreement "can and should be interpreted and implemented . . . to protect public health and, in partic-ular, to promote access to medicines for all."[42] The Doha Declaration was also complemented by the WTO "August 30th decision" in 2003, aimed at allowing the export of generics to other developing countries. The new Global Fund and US President's Emergency Plan for AIDS Relief (PEPFAR) (see chapters 7 and 8) accelerated expansion of anti-retroviral generics in the developing world, and 95% of global donor-funded antiretrovirals were generics by 2008.[41]

Despite these frameworks and advancements, when a new gold-standard triple therapy for HIV entered the market in 2018, it cost $75 a year in many African nations and $39,000 a year in the United States, exemplifying practical challenges that remain to balancing the TRIPS tug-of-war.[43] HIV drug development is evolving, and price cuts are brought about by a competitive market, which has not developed to the extent needed to make HIV drugs affordable in the United States. This is possible in part because almost no one taking antiretrovirals in the United States is paying directly for them. Instead, entities like Medicare,

Medicaid, and the Ryan White HIV/AIDS Program shell out enormous sums to drug companies. The country spends an estimated $20 billion annually on HIV medications, constituting the largest item in Medicaid's drug budget.[43] No other diseases have such drug-payment programs.

Sofosbuvir and Patent Implications

Another side of the TRIPS patent protection coin is illustrated by sofosbuvir. Sofosbuvir (brand name Sovaldi) received US Food and Drug Administration approval in 2013 and offered a major improvement in hepatitis C treatment. Sofosbuvir has a 3- to 6-month treatment window and a 90% cure rate, compared to the previously standard 6 to 12 months of medications with severe side effects and a cure rate around 70%. It was also the first oral treatment regimen available, replacing daily injections. With exclusive manufacturing rights for 16 years, made possible through US IP protection policies, a course of the medication in the United States currently costs $84,000.[44,45] The drug's hefty price tag is in sharp contrast to estimates that the cost to manufacture a course is only $101.[46]

Sofosbuvir renewed discussion about what level of innovation merits IP protection; the compounds used in the drug were adaptations from existing HIV and cancer medications, with one adjustment. Almost as soon as the drug hit the market, patent challenges ensued. In the United States, the Initiative for Medicines, Access, and Knowledge (I-MAK) filed challenges, arguing that the patents did not "meet the legal standards for novelty and non-obviousness."[47] Civil society organizations from 17 countries in Europe similarly opposed the patent over the lack of inventiveness. When the patent was upheld by the European Patent Office, six organizations, including Médecins Sans Frontières (Doctors Without Borders), appealed the decision because it did not "meet the requirements to be a patentable invention from a legal or scientific perspective."[45] In the United Kingdom, where the patents were upheld, the National Health Service delayed its introduction in light of its extraordinarily high cost ($53,500 for a course of the medication in 2015).[48]

India's patent laws have a higher threshold for innovation than those in the United States and the United Kingdom, requiring developers to prove that they have made a significant scientific advancement; minor improvements to existing drugs are not considered patentable. India's patent department deemed Gilead's innovation with sofosbuvir to be insufficient for patenting and rejected the applications, causing Gilead to shift to a nonexclusive agreement with generic producers.[49] Seven Indian manufacturers received the full rights to independently produce the drug and the ability to set their own prices—landing on about $8 per pill compared to the US cost of $1,000 per pill.[50,51]

Sofosbuvir's patent process in China was more convoluted. Concerned that Gilead had acquired the knowledge for the sofosbuvir medication through prior public research, China's patent board rejected Gilead's patent just as India did. However, to become more competitive in global trade agreements, China had adopted data-exclusivity provisions that protected Gilead's data for six years, even though the sofosbuvir patent was ultimately rejected. It is estimated that it will take five to seven years to become available in the Chinese market and will still cost between $15,000 and $20,000, inaccessible to most of the population, with its GDP per capita of $12,500.[52]

Demand for the drug has been universal, though access to it is not, leading to the proliferation of medical tourism to India. One Shanghai-based company offers a four-day package tour to New Delhi, including doctor's appointments, medications, flights, hotels, and even a half-day tour of the city.[53] Despite efforts, like the Doha Declaration, to advance public health priorities through trade-related policies like TRIPS, drug pricing and availability continue to perpetuate global inequality.

Pharmaceutical management is complicated at every step; drug discovery, approval, manufacturing, pricing, efficacy, and resistance all threaten to challenge progress in global disease management. Learning to balance competing forces in public health, economics, and national security will be paramount to success in global health pharmaceuticals.

Concluding Thoughts
BILL FOEGE

On Pharmaceuticals

Pharmaceuticals provide a positive case for globalism. Remoteness no longer precludes benefiting from cutting-edge science. New experiments on government support of vaccine and drug development and distribution during COVID-19, joint programs by various companies and the Bill & Melinda Gates Foundation, and consortiums such as Gavi (Global Alliance for Vaccines and Immunization) all provide hope that global health responses are improving. Leadership in global health is not defined by a title, but rather by the people who are able to organize effective coalitions.

On Bioterrorism

Lessons must be continuously studied and refined. They require maintenance. Promoting maintenance is a thankless job, but essential. Let's look at one example from CDC history.

The frightening challenge of bioterrorism requires a defensive plan against every known agent that could potentially be used by a terrorist. It requires a system for deploying such a counteraction and the resources and personnel to manage that system. It requires surveillance systems to detect the presence of such agents, and it requires a mechanism to quickly identify organisms not seen before.

In the early 1990s, the CDC began developing such a defense. A systematic review of agents that could be used was undertaken. Those scientists most familiar with each organism worked on scenarios that might be used to spread it; then a defense plan was developed for each organism.

The CDC worked with the FBI as the approaches became more complex. This resulted in developing a secure phone system and a secure room so that discussions could be held with the FBI that could not be intercepted by third parties.

Stuart Kingma was in charge of organizing the defense plan. A careful, even obsessive planner, he oversaw the development of the defense and, with others, continued to seek weak spots that needed strengthening. He organized a call schedule, so that there would be 24/7 coverage to take calls, alert the appropriate people, and initiate a reaction team to work in the secure room.

However, the weak spots may be in places not anticipated. A new director was appointed to be head of the CDC. In due time, he was briefed on bioterrorism, the system to confront it, and what it could do. His surprising reaction was to say, "That problem will never happen." He dismantled the program.

Years later, when anthrax was deliberately distributed by a domestic terrorist, the response team had long been disbanded and the response, while appropriate, lacked the speed and vigor possible. The CDC did not use the plans that had been developed.

The lesson is that the world still needs robust plans at the national and global level to respond to bioterrorist threats. The best thinking should be gathered, and response programs funded and staffed as we would a fire department. No matter how long the gap between fires, the response must always be ready. This requires superb, but often neglected, maintenance.

CHAPTER 15

Promoting Positive Change

BILL FOEGE

During my lifetime, one striking change in the field of global health has been the increased attention it's getting. When I became interested in this area 70 years ago, it was difficult to find mentors. One teacher said a career in global health should be approached knowing that there would be no major change in health outcomes in my lifetime and that the work would be in providing a foundation for changes in the next generation. It would be like planting a tree that would only provide shade for the next generation.

This prediction turned out to be far from the truth. One human disease, smallpox, has now been eliminated. One animal disease, rinderpest (which has implications for human health, as many people depend on milk and meat from cattle), has been eradicated. With attention being given to tuberculosis, malaria, cholera, and other diseases, many missed the fact that measles was the biggest killer of all, with over 3 million deaths per year. Morbidity and mortality from measles is now a fraction of earlier numbers. Polio, at this writing, has been reduced to small areas in a handful of countries, sparing thousands from death and paralysis each year. Guinea worm disease is in its final chapter.

While the once common childhood diseases of pertussis, diphtheria, and rubella no longer constitute the threats they once posed, even cervical cancer and liver cancer deaths, major causes of mortality, have been declining because of human papillomavirus and hepatitis vaccines. The CDC reports that, in the Southeast Asia region, hepatitis B vaccination prevented approximately 16 million chronic infections and 2.6 million related deaths during 1992–2015. Similarly, in the Western Pacific region, vaccination prevented over 37 million chronic infections and 7 million deaths among children born between 1990 and 2014. Likewise, cervical cancer, the other cancer with a vaccine, is also showing a reduction in deaths. Thus, two good vaccines are showing an impact on cancer but are being underused. No woman in this country should die of cervical cancer, yet it still happens 10 times a day. The challenge to use our tools is a management challenge rather than a scientific challenge. Good science provides the best answers; good management provides the best results.

Vaccines have become the foundation of global health and will continue to be so. We expect vaccines to emerge for other infectious diseases, cancers, and perhaps even alcohol and drug cravings, as well as heart disease. (Vaccine resistance, however, has made clear that the barrier to better health and vaccine use is not just nature, but also *human* nature.)

But the good news doesn't end. Even diseases once considered to be the problems of poor countries—such as onchocerciasis (river blindness), trachoma, lymphatic filariasis, roundworms, hookworms, and schistosomiasis—are receding as threats. These accomplishments are all because of organized programs that incorporate health workers, corporations, governments, and nongovernmental organizations.

In my lifetime, global health workers were often criticized for spending money on problems that would never be conquered. Now it is clear that life expectancy is improving everyplace, not by chance but because of organized global health efforts. (Nevertheless, while averages may improve, the lot of the bottom quartile has barely moved. The challenge in global health is found in changing standard deviations, not simply in changing averages.)

Another surprise has been the interest of young people to enter the field. I was told if I wanted to pursue global health as a career, I would need to create my own path. The success of smallpox eradication provided a hope for those with global health interests. However, it was the involvement of the Gates family, at the turn of the century, that suddenly multiplied opportunities for clinical practice, research, and public programs to speed up the goal of global health equity and provide pathways to global public health.

Disparities in Global Health

Yet the progress is uneven. The picture is one of both breathtaking improvements and breathtaking disparities. The poorest people in every country are still spectators to the great changes. And such indices as maternal mortality in Africa or Afghanistan—and even Atlanta—are an embarrassment to our sense of justice and to our belief in our creative abilities to solve problems.

While the progress in infectious disease control is heartening, the limitations in approaching chronic conditions—including heart disease, strokes, alcohol and drug use, diabetes, and obesity—are sobering. To make it worse, these problems are actually exploding in poor countries. Yet many leaders and politicians involved in resource allocation still do not regard these as public health problems.

Making Eye Contact with the Future

Young people going into global health fields have job security. Good. Because there is so much to be done.

A major concern in global health is population growth. At one time, global health critics argued that population growth was the result of global health successes. That turned out to be false. The fastest population growth rates over the past decades have been in the countries with the highest death rates, such as African countries. Disease has not been an efficient way of reducing population growth. But give people the opportunity to control their own fertility, and they are eager to do so.

Even religious beliefs opposing birth control cannot discourage the use of contraception, once it is available. The lowest birth rates were soon seen in Italy, France, and other Catholic countries. But the inability of the poorest people in the poorest countries to use contraception has permitted rapid population growth.

The twin problems of population growth and increasing consumption of resources have led to the current emergency of climate change. Even as population growth slows, resource consumption per person increases.

Global health workers of today need to enter fields beyond the traditional concerns, to reduce poverty and production of carbon dioxide, methane, and other climate-changing products. This means that no subject that can affect human well-being should be viewed as beyond the interest and concern of global health workers. It also means that every global health worker must be a generalist and specialist simultaneously. A generalist to understand as much as possible about how the world operates and the interconnections of knowledge. A specialist to have a skill to change the massive overall problems of the world. While daunting, this means that, for the foreseeable future, global health will continue to be one of the most exciting of all vocational fields.

The expectations were great for those involved in smallpox and polio eradication, measles control, Guinea worm eradication, and river blindness reduction. These workers were undaunted by the frequent opinions that their goal could not be met. Now, the world needs global health workers who have the vision and tenacity to address even larger problems. Smallpox-eradication lessons are presented on the website *9Lessons.org*. Examples cited there show that these lessons are not confined to smallpox or even public health. They are life lessons to becoming better ancestors. What we do to improve life quality now is exceedingly important, but it is dwarfed by the contributions we can make to the future by becoming better ancestors.

The Changing Teaching Agenda

The agenda for global health teaching may change in two significant ways. The first will be with the curriculum itself, and the second will be in the approach to teaching.

Future Curricula

Given the above comments, the curriculum will be based on how to prevent premature mortality and unnecessary morbidity, and how to improve the quality of life. Public health training will still concentrate on developing skills in epidemiology and statistics, but it will broaden to include the entire range of infectious diseases, chronic diseases, intentional and unintentional injuries, mental health disorders, and the environment. Training will also include tracking risk factors and protective factors from genomic surveillance and tracking health outcomes to determine optimal ways of delivering the increasing knowledge and technologies becoming available. Finally, global health teaching will include grounding in political science to incorporate politics and global health in seamless approaches to problem-solving.

Included skills will be helping students to become better communicators. Science gets its power only when used. Public health workers need to be better translators of their knowledge to the general public so that the public can partner in the use of science. No matter how good and miraculous coronavirus vaccines became, they had very little power to directly help the people refusing to take them. Vaccine deniers become unwitting threats to themselves and to others. (And if they are a risk to themselves and others, should this be included in the International Classification of Diseases [IDC] code? This certainly has moral implications and places a burden on public health providers and communicators.)

The Future Approach to Teaching

The approach to teaching will also change. Schools of public health have always had three objectives: to impart a philosophy, provide skills, and transfer knowledge. A major portion of the time in training was the transfer of knowledge. Lectures, note-taking, questions and answers, and testing were part of the routine.

A major change has taken place in recent decades, however. Knowledge is now readily available without a trip to the library. Much of the knowledge transfer in the past was already outdated by the time students went into practice. The goal now should be training students (and later practitioners) how to gather and evaluate knowledge, with far less time devoted to lectures or other forms of knowledge transfer.

This shift would allow more time for the practicing of skills development and, crucially, in the nurturing of a philosophy. Students cannot predict the opportunities that they will be presented with in the future. Therefore, *a life philosophy is far more important than a life plan*. A life plan is based on what is known now, and that will not be the world students encounter.

A philosophy is best transferred by means of respected and accomplished mentors. Mentorship is one criterion that predicts postgraduation success of students. The best mentors continue to have influence for years, and that is now possible through telecommunication, even for students from other countries.

What should be included in a global health philosophy? Three ingredients seem crucial. The first is to instill the idea of getting the science right. While many people have a fear of science, Thomas Huxley described science as, "common sense at its best." Most people regard themselves as having common sense.

The second ingredient was described by historian Will Durant, who said the first scientist known by name was Imhotep. He was a scientist, a physician, and the artist who designed the Step Pyramid. Durant pointed out that this melding of art and science is a combination that should be sought as it combines the structure of science with the creativity of art, and it leads to "creative common sense at its best."

A third component in a global health philosophy was demonstrated by Roger Bacon, 800 years ago. He was asked to do a summary of science for the Pope. Bacon, a visionary scientist who predicted cars, planes, and submarines, told the Pope that science lacked a moral compass. This requires training scientists to have a moral compass. Developing these three ingredients—common sense at its best, creativity, and a moral compass—provides "moral, creative common sense at its best." This is a worthy goal of schools of public health. But it is a goal that would require schools to find the best mentors possible and create ways to provide every student with such a mentor.

Mentorship is the core of global health training. It provides students the opportunity to observe their teachers, to learn about their beliefs, their philosophy, their approach to life, and their treatment of peers, patients, and students. In short, mentors provide the chance for students to copy role models.

Another predictor of success following graduation is the use of tools and skills under the supervision of experienced practitioners. This is often an internship or a problem-solving period in another culture. Every school should make this opportunity available. To become a pediatrician, it is not sufficient to read about pediatrics. The resident must actually take care of sick children. Likewise, to become a surgeon it is necessary to perform increasingly more difficult surgical procedures. Schools of public health could offer academic positions to local and state health officers and incorporate experiences for students to actually take responsibility for portions of local public health practice. It might be possible to incorporate this hands-on experience with mentorship, providing students with fulfilling practices that would better prepare them for postgraduation activities.

The Lessons of the *Vasa*

Mark Rosenberg, president and CEO of the Task Force for Global Health from 2000 to 2016, tells a haunting story that reminds us of the importance of not forgetting hard-learned lessons:

> In the 1600s, Sweden was fighting invaders from across the sea, to little avail. Finally, the king decided on a way to beat them. They would build a three-deck ship, loaded with cannons on each deck. Named the *Vasa*, the ship took three years to build in an area near Stockholm. It was one of the largest and most expensive ships in the world. When it was finally completed, huge celebrations were planned for the day the ship sailed out of the canal near Stockholm. But the ship tipped over and sank on its maiden voyage; it took only

20 minutes to totally sink—it was just too heavy. All the families who were present to celebrate watched the ship sink. It was a horrific event. What was supposed to be a celebration was a tragedy.

And yet no one in the rest of the world—and, indeed, in Sweden, itself—knew about this tragedy until the 1950s, when a few fishermen were fishing along the canal where the *Vasa* sailed and pulled up some wooden railings. Explorers went down and looked, and lo and behold, it was the *Vasa*. The explorers hadn't known what it was.

"Why didn't they know?" Rosenberg asked in a recent Contagious Conversations podcast.[1] "People forgot. They forgot about the *Vasa*."

In the early 2000s, Rosenberg visited the site of the *Vasa*'s tragic sinking. He asked someone, in what is now the Vasa Museum, how the town could have forgotten such a tragic event. The man said, "Whenever anything happens, there's only three generations that remember: the generation that did it, their sons and their daughters, and their grandchildren. After three generations, it's forgotten. This happened to the *Vasa*, and it will happen to you."

The lesson of the *Vasa* was not lost for those in global health, particularly the smallpox warriors. "Eradicating smallpox was the Holy Grail of global health," said Rosenberg. "It was the most important, most spectacular global health achievement ever. And the lessons learned from it needed to be remembered."[1]

Becoming Better Ancestors and *9Lessons.org*

It was out of a belief that the public health world did not want the lessons of the smallpox-eradication effort to be similarly forgotten, that, in December 2022, the Center for Global Health Innovation announced the launch of Becoming Better Ancestors. This project is committed to solving global health challenges and creating positive change for future generations.

Jonas Salk introduced me to the idea of becoming better ancestors. It was the title of a talk he gave in the Nehru lecture decades ago. He

LESSON 1: THIS IS A CAUSE & EFFECT WORLD.	LESSON 2: KNOW, SHARE, & ACT ON THE TRUTH.	LESSON 3: COALITIONS ARE ESSENTIAL.
LESSON 4: AVOID CERTAINTY.	LESSON 5: BUILD IN EVALUATION & IMPROVEMENT.	LESSON 6: RESPECT THE CULTURE. CULTURE MATTERS.
LESSON 7: SEEK STRONG LEADERSHIP & MANAGEMENT.	LESSON 8: MOBILIZE POLITICAL WILL.	LESSON 9: MOVE TOWARDS GLOBAL HEALTH EQUITY.

The nine lessons learned from the successful smallpox-eradication campaign. These lessons are not confined to smallpox or even public health. They are life lessons for becoming better ancestors.
Source: Becoming Better Ancestors team and the Task Force for Global Health, Inc.

said, "It's important to be a good citizen. We all should try to do that, but it's even more important to be a good ancestor."

The first project of Becoming Better Ancestors was a website—*9Lessons.org*—to introduce people to the major lessons from the smallpox campaign. The site also has a series and curriculum, called Nine Lessons to Change the World. The curriculum focuses on nine simple, proven, and reliable ways to approach global health threats.

There are many lessons from smallpox eradication. I suppose we could name a hundred. But we selected nine that are so important, and that go beyond smallpox, beyond public health, to life in general. I put them in three categories.

The first category contains basic lessons that everyone knows—lessons that help us build intentionally.

> *Lesson 1: This is a cause-and-effect world. If we understand the causes, we can change the effects.*

This is not a world of magic. There are reasons why things happen. In global health, we try to figure out what those reasons are, so we know how to prevent them in the future.

Lesson 2: Know the truth. Share the truth. Act on the truth.
This is obviously related to the fact that it's a cause-and-effect world. There are so many times that I did not want to know the truth because it was so overwhelming. I can remember that, in India, the first search for smallpox cases that we had of villages, we didn't expect to find many cases. It was a low point of transmission. But in six days, we found 10,000 new cases of smallpox that no one knew about. Imagine if we had not sought to know the truth?

Lesson 3: Coalitions are essential.
We can't do anything alone. This is an old lesson. Polybius taught us this 2,000 years ago.

   Then there is a category of three lessons that cause us to pause and reflect.

Lesson 4: Avoid certainty.
The physicist Richard Feynman made this principle so clear. "Physics is the most certain of sciences, and we're not certain," he wrote. "It's a shame that politicians and theologians may be so certain they try to prove that they're right. But in science, we have to avoid certainty. It's the Achilles heel of science."

Lesson 5: Build in consequential evaluation and continuous improvement.
Given that we're *not* certain, we need to evaluate to learn what is really happening, rather than what we *hoped* would happen, and then continuously improve as we find out what is going on.

Lesson 6: Respect the culture.
This is the final lesson in this category. *Culture matters.* If you try to fight culture, you will always lose. Unfortunately, it's

something we often learn in retrospect ("I wish I hadn't done that").

When we've learned these six lessons, we need to summon the courage to go to scale.

Lesson 7: Seek strong leadership and management.
This means combining science and management. Science gives us the best answers. Management gives us the best results. How do we put those two together?

Lesson 8: Mobilize political will.
With political will, anything is possible; without it, nothing is. Oftentimes, in public health, we are upset with a political decision. But we need to recognize that we're totally dependent on politicians. They're the ones who provide us with the resources. We have to get them invested in the outcomes, so that they're not just funding us, they're funding an outcome that they have already bought into.

Lesson 9: The best solutions move us closer to global health equity.
Move toward a global solution. Every place is both local and global. Therefore, any place you're doing public health, you're doing global public health. The objective is to get global health equity.

If you scroll through the table of contents for this book, I hope you'll see that the failures and successes researched and reported here reflect the value of and need for these nine lessons.

The Hope for Global Health Equity

British historian Arnold Toynbee predicted we would end the 20th century closing the gap on health equity. It did not happen. However, the improvement in tools, the increase in resources, the age of instantaneous communications, and the demonstration that it is possible to reach global goals all portend a future that could achieve global health equity in the lifetime of our children.

Many people don't feel that polio, onchocerciasis, or lymphatic filariasis are threats to them or their families. Yet the world was able to organize to reduce these threats. With this experience, we need to be bold in approaching a spectrum of threats that can affect everyone: climate change, nuclear weapons, the potential threat of synthetic biology, and artificial intelligence. To these generally accepted threats to human existence, we must now consider social media as an additional threat. What it has done to civilized discourse is cause for great concern.

Making eye contact with the future is an essential ingredient in public health education. Tenacity is required because, as the late Surgeon General Leonard Scheele said, "The world cannot be allowed to exist half healthy and half sick."[2] We must live up to the description of Harlan Cleveland, who said that what fueled global health workers was "unwarranted optimism." *That* is what made it possible for them to do impossible things.

Our Proxy

When I think of becoming a good ancestor, what I see in my mind are the faces of children 300 years from now, trying to get my attention—because they've given me their proxy. They're pleading, "Please make the best decisions you can for us." It's easy for us to make a good decision for ourselves and for our family, for our loved ones. But time and space put us in a difficult position to make good decisions for a child 300 years from now.

That's what we need to think of, that we have their proxy. We have so much power because of that proxy, but we have to use it well.

WILLIAM H. FOEGE, MD, MPH, is Emeritus Presidential Distinguished Professor of International Health at Emory University and an early consultant to the Bill & Melinda Gates Foundation. He is the author of *House on Fire: The Fight to Eradicate Smallpox* and *The Fears of the Rich, The Needs of the Poor: My Years at the CDC*. In 2012, he was awarded the Presidential Medal of Freedom.

PAUL ELISH, MPH, is currently pursuing a PhD in International Health at Johns Hopkins University. He holds an MPH in Global Epidemiology from Emory University and most recently worked in international respiratory virus surveillance strengthening at the Centers for Disease Control and Prevention. His prior work experience spans the academic, private, and nonprofit sectors, with a primary focus on public health issues in Latin America, Sub-Saharan Africa, and the United States.

ALISON T. HOOVER, MPH, is a researcher at Emory University focusing on gender, reproductive and sexual health, and bioethics. Prior to Emory, she worked as a communications consultant in Vietnam and a program evaluator in Mexico and Bolivia. She was named a 120 Under 40 global leader in family planning by the William H. Gates Sr. Institute for Population and Reproductive Health in 2019.

MADISON GABRIELLA LEE, MPH, is a research environmental scientist. Her research is focused on assessing exposure to chemical contaminants and has appeared in the *International Journal of Hygiene and Environmental Health*. She is an alumna of North Carolina State University and the Rollins School of Public Health at Emory University.

DEBORAH CHEN TSENG, MPH, is a current Oak Ridge Institute for Science and Education (ORISE) fellow with CDC-INFO at the Centers for Disease Control and Prevention. She previously worked in Appalachian Kentucky with middle schoolers, high schoolers, and staff in the areas of health education and health promotion.

KIERA CHAN, MPH, is a PhD student at the University of Alabama at Birmingham. Her research studies the intersection of patient-centered care and health disparities, and her work has been featured in scientific publications on women's health and in a TEDx Talk. She has worked previously with several nonprofits, including Days for Girls International, CARE International, and the International Association for Premenstrual Disorders. She is committed to global health through community work, advocacy, and research.

TOM PAULSON is a journalist based in Seattle specializing in science, medicine, and global development. He has a BS in chemistry from Pacific Lutheran University and an MA in science writing from Johns Hopkins University. He has worked for the *Seattle Post-Intelligencer* and NPR affiliate KNKX and was also executive editor for the online news site *Humanosphere*.

Chapter 2. Politics and Global Health

1. McGinnis JM, Foege WH. Actual causes of death in the United States. JAMA. 1993 Nov 110;270(18):2207–12.
2. Foege WH, Amler RW, White CC. Closing the gap: report of the Carter Center Health Policy Consultation. JAMA. 1985 Sept 13; 254(10):1355–58.
3. Carter J, Carter R. Everything to gain: making the most of the rest of your life. New York: Random House; 1987.
4. WHO Collaborating Center for Dracunculiasis Eradication. The death of Gary Strieker. CDC Subject: GUINEA WORM WRAP-UP #290.
5. Foul water/fiery serpent (2010), https://www.imdb.com/title /tt1620740/.
6. Barney GO, editor. The Global 2000 report to the President of the U.S.: entering the 21st century. Vol l: The summary report. New York: Pergamon Press; 1900.
7. The church's challenge in health. https://www.cartercenter.org/resources /pdfs/pdf-archive/thechurchschallengeinhealth-10251989.pdf.
8. Faith and health. https://www.cartercenter.org/resources/pdfs/pdf -archive/faithanfhealth-10011998.pdf.

Chapter 3. The Legacy of Colonialism in Global Health

1. Popkin JD. A concise history of the Haitian revolution. Somerset, NJ: John Wiley & Sons; 2021.
2. Geggus D. The naming of Haiti. New West Indian Guide/Nieuwe West-Indische Gids. 1997;71(1–2):43–68.
3. Higman BW. A concise history of the Caribbean. Cambridge: Cambridge University Press; 2010.
4. Arnold D. Warm climates and western medicine: the emergence of tropical medicine, 1500–1900. Leiden (NL): Brill; 2020.
5. Alchon SA. A pest in the land: new world epidemics in a global perspective. Albuquerque: University of New Mexico Press; 2003.

6. Chippaux J-P, Chippaux A. Yellow fever in Africa and the Americas: a historical and epidemiological perspective. J Venom Anim Toxins Incl Trop Dis. 2018;24.

7. Webb JL. Humanity's burden: a global history of malaria. New York: Cambridge University Press; 2009.

8. Grandmaison OLC. L'Empire des hygiénistes: faire vivre aux colonies. Paris: Fayard; 2014.

9. Öberg S, Rönnbäck K. Mortality among European settlers in pre-colonial West Africa: The "White Man's Grave" revisited. 2016. No 20, Göteborg Papers in Economic History, University of Gothenburg, Unit for Economic History. https://econpapers.repec.org /scripts/getreflist.pl?h=repec%3Ahhs%3Agunhis%3A0020;reflist =citec;pg=1.

10. Johnson R, Khalid A. Public health in the British Empire: intermediaries, subordinates, and the practice of public health, 1850–1960. New York: Routledge; 2012.

11. Cook G. Tropical medicine: an illustrated history of the pioneers. Amsterdam (NL): Elsevier; 2007.

12. Harrison M. Public health in British India: Anglo-Indian preventive medicine 1859–1914. Cambridge: Cambridge University Press; 1994.

13. Halvorson SJ, Wescoat Jr JL. Guarding the sons of empire: military–state–society relations in water, sanitation and health programs of mid-19th-century India. Water. 2020;12(2):429.

14. Teixeira LA, Pimenta TS, Hochman G, editors. História da saúde no Brasil. Sao Paulo: Hucitec Editora; 2018.

15. Risse G. History of Western Medicine from Hippocrates to germ theory. In: Risse GB. The Cambridge world history of human disease. Cambridge: Cambridge University Press; 1993:11–19.

16. Worboys M. Was there a bacteriological revolution in late nineteenth-century medicine? Stud Hist Philos Biol Biomed Sci. 2007;38(1):20–42.

17. Loudon I. Western medicine: an illustrated history. Oxford: Oxford University Press; 1997.

18. Huber V. The unification of the globe by disease? The international sanitary conferences on cholera, 1851–1894. Hist J. 2006;49(2):453–76.

19. Headrick DR. Sleeping sickness epidemics and colonial responses in East and Central Africa, 1900–1940. PLoS Negl Trop Dis. 2014;8(4):e2772.

20. Lyons M. Public health in colonial Africa: the Belgian Congo. In: The history of public health and the modern state. Clio Medica vol. 26. Leiden (NL): Brill; 1994:356–84.
21. Stahl RM. The economics of starvation: laissez-faire ideology and famine in Colonial India. In: Thorup M, editor. Intellectual history of economic normativities; 2016:169–84. https://link.springer.com /book/10.1057/978-1-137-59416-7.
22. Naono A. Burmese health officers in the transformation of public health in Colonial Burma in the 1920s and 1930s. In: Johnson R, Khalid A. Public health in the British Empire: intermediaries, subordinates, and the practice of public health, 1850–1960. New York: Routledge; 2012:126–42.
23. Johnson R. Mantsemei, interpreters, and the successful eradication of plague: the 1908 plague epidemic in Colonial Accra. In: Johnson R, Khalid A. Public health in the British Empire: intermediaries, subordinates, and the practice of public health, 1850–1960. New York: Routledge; 2012:135–53.
24. Khalid A. "Unscientific and insanitary": hereditary sweepers and customary rights in the United Provinces. In: Johnson R, Khalid A. Public health in the British Empire: intermediaries, subordinates, and the practice of public health, 1850–1960. New York: Routledge; 2012:51–70.
25. Lang S. The control of birth: pupil midwives in nineteenth-century Madras. In: Johnson R, Khalid A. Public health in the British Empire: intermediaries, subordinates, and the practice of public health, 1850–1960. New York: Routledge; 2012:32–50.
26. Kalusa W. Medical training, African auxiliaries, and social healing in colonial Mwinilunga, Northern Rhodesia (Zambia), 1945–1964. In: Johnson R, Khalid A. Public health in the British Empire: intermediaries, subordinates, and the practice of public health, 1850–1960. New York: Routledge; 2012:154–70.
27. Pearson JL. The colonial politics of global health: France and the United Nations in postwar Africa. Cambridge, MA: Harvard University Press; 2018.

Chapter 4. Militaries and Global Health

1. Anderson W. Colonial pathologies: American tropical medicine, race, and hygiene in the Philippines. Durham, NC: Duke University Press; 2006.

2. Cook GC. Tropical medicine an illustrated history of the pioneers. London: Academic Press; 2007.
3. Osborne MA. The emergence of tropical medicine in France. Chicago: University of Chicago Press; 2014.
4. Becker C, Collignon R. Épidémies et médecine coloniale en Afrique de l'Ouest. Cahiers d'études et de recherches francophones/Santé. 1999;8(6):411–16.
5. Bienia RA, Stein E, Bienia BH. United States Public Health Service Hospitals (1798–1981)—the end of an era. Waltham, MA: Mass Medical Society; 1983:166–68.
6. Commissioned Corps of the U.S. Public Health Service. Our history. 2021; Available from: https://www.usphs.gov/history.
7. Grandmaison OLC. L'Empire des hygiénistes: Faire vivre aux colonies. Paris: Fayard; 2014.
8. Lederer SE. Walter Reed and the yellow fever experiments. The Oxford textbook of clinical research ethics. Oxford: Oxford University Press; 2008:9–17.
9. Minna Stern A. Yellow fever crusade: US colonialism, tropical medicine, and the international politics of mosquito control, 1900–1920. In: Bashford A, editor. Medicine at the border: disease, globalization and security, 1850 to the present. London: Palgrave Macmillan; 2006.
10. Etheridge EW. Sentinel for health: a history of the Centers for Disease Control. Berkeley: University of California Press; 1992.
11. Thacker SB, Dannenberg AL, Hamilton DH. Epidemic intelligence service of the Centers for Disease Control and Prevention: 50 years of training and service in applied epidemiology. Am J Epidemiol. 2001;154(11):985–92.
12. Michaud J, Moss K, Licina D, Waldman R, Kamradt-Scott A, Bartee M, et al. Militaries and global health: peace, conflict, and disaster response. Lancet. 2019:393(10168):276–86.
13. Gordon S. Health, stabilization and securitization: towards understanding the drivers of the military role in health interventions. Med Confl Surv. 2011;27(1):43–66.
14. Osterholm MT. Global health security—an unfinished journey. Emerg Infect Dis. 2017;23(Suppl 1):S225.
15. Global Health Security Agenda. Global Health Security agenda. [cited 2023 April 7]; Available from: https://globalhealthsecurity agenda.org/.

Chapter 5. Religious Missions and Global Health

1. Afshar A, Steensma DP, Kyle RA. Albert Schweitzer: humanitarian with a "reverence for life." Mayo Clinic Proc. 2019;94(7):e91–92. https://doi.org/10.1016/j.mayocp.2019.05.009.
2. Centre de Recherches Médicales de Lambaréné. https://www.cermel .org/history.php. Accessed February 14, 2021.
3. Dr. Schweitzer's Hospital Fund (UK) - Schweitzer's Hospital in Lambaréné; 2016 Nov 18. https://web.archive.org/web /20161118195234/http://www.schweitzershospitalfund.org.uk /lambarene.html. Accessed February 14, 2021.
4. Baron D, Mullins L. Historic Albert Schweitzer Hospital adapts to new Africa. The World from PRX. https://www.pri.org/stories/2012 -05-17/historic-albert-schweitzer-hospital-adapts-new-africa. Accessed February 14, 2021.
5. Chesterman CC. Medical missions in Belgian Congo. Int Rev Mission. 1937;26(3):378–85.
6. Northrup D. A church in search of a state: Catholic missions in Eastern Zaire, 1879–1930. J Church State. 1988;30(2):309–19. https://www.jstor.org/stable/23917546.
7. Au S. Medical orders: Catholic and Protestant missionary medicine in the Belgian Congo 1880–1940. BMGN-LCHR. 2017;132(1):62. https://doi.org/10.18352/bmgn-lchr.10309.
8. Joseph DG. "Essentially Christian, eminently philanthropic": the mission to lepers in British India. História, Ciências, Saúde Man-guinhos. 2003;10(Suppl l):247–75. https://doi.org/10.1590/S0104 -59702003000400012.
9. Mkenda F. A Protestant verdict on the Jesuit missionary approach in Africa: David Livingstone and memories of the early Jesuit presence in South Central Africa. In: Mkenda F, Maryks RA, editors. Encounters between Jesuits and Protestants in Africa. 13:59–80. Brill; 2018. http://www.jstor.org/stable/10.1163/j .ctvbqs62t.6.
10. African Religious Health Assets Programme. Appreciating assets: the contribution of religion to universal access in Africa. Geneva: WHO; 2006.
11. Kagawa RC, Anglemyer A, Montagu D. The scale of faith based organization participation in health service delivery in developing countries: systemic review and meta-analysis. PLoS One. 2012;7(11). https://doi.org/10.1371/journal.pone.0048457.

12. Dilger H. Claiming territory: medical mission, interreligious revivalism, and the spatialization of health interventions in urban Tanzania. Med Anthropol. 2014;33(1):52–67. https://doi.org/10.1080/01459740.2013.821987.

13. Hajar R. The pulse in ancient medicine Part 1. Heart Views. 2018 Jan-Mar;19(1):36–43. https://doi.org/10.4103/HEARTVIEWS.HEARTVIEWS_23_18.

14. Gulick EV. Peter Parker and the opening of China. Cambridge (MA): Harvard University Press; 1973.

15. Ghasemzadeh N, Zafari AM. A brief journey into the history of the arterial pulse. Cardiol Res Pract. 2011. https://doi.org/10.4061/2011/164832.

16. Parker, Peter (1804–1888): medical missionary in China. https://www.bu.edu/missiology/missionary-biography/n-o-p-q/parker-peter-1804-1888/. Accessed March 12, 2021.

17. Mohammadpour M, Abrishami M, Masoumi A, Hashemi H. Trachoma: past, present and future. J Curr Ophthalmol. 2016 Sep 19;28(4):165–69. https://doi.org/10.1016/j.joco.2016.08.011.

18. Bowers JZ. The founding of Peking Union Medical College: policies and personalities. Bull Hist Med. 1971;45(4):305–21.

19. Welter B. She hath done what she could: Protestant women's missionary careers in nineteenth-century America. Am Q. 1978 winter;30(5):624–38.

20. Chawla Singh M. Gender, religion, and the heathen lands: American missionary women in South Asia (1860s–1940s). London: Taylor and Francis Group, Routledge; 1999.

21. Nalini M. Pioneer woman physician as medical missionary to the women of the Orient: Clara A. Swain, M.D. (1834–1910). Int J Innov Manag Technol. 2010;1(2). http://www.ijimt.org/papers/27-C322.pdf. Accessed March 4, 2021.

22. CMC Vellore. https://www.cmch-vellore.edu/2col.aspx?ptype=CONTENT&pid=P171127016%20&mid=M171127123. Accessed January 9, 2021.

23. Dries A. "Fire and flame": Anna Dengel and the Medical Mission to Women and Children. Missiology. 1999;27(4):495–501. https://doi.org/10.1177/009182969902700408.

24. Johnson L, Wall BM. Women, religion, and maternal health care in Ghana, 1945–2000: Fam Community Health. 2014 Jul-Sep;37(3):223–30. https://doi.org/10.1097/FCH.0000000000000032.

25. Dries A. Hospitality as a life stance in mission: elements from Catholic mission experience in the twentieth century. Int Bull Mission Res. 2015;39(4):194–97. https://doi.org/10.1177/2396939315039 00407.

26. Jacob JT, Franco-Paredes C. The stigmatization of leprosy in India and its impact on future approaches to elimination and control. PLoS Negl Trop Dis. 2008;2(1). https://doi.org/10.1371/journal.pntd.0000113.

27. Worboys M. The colonial world as mission and mandate: leprosy and empire, 1900–1940. Osiris. 2000;15:207–18.

28. Vongsathorn K. Gnawing pains, festering ulcers, and nightmare suffering: selling leprosy as a humanitarian cause in the British Empire, c. 1890–1960. J Imp Commonw Hist. 2012;40(5):863–78. https://doi.org/10.1080/03086534.2012.730839.

29. Nash JE. Paul Wilson Brand. BMJ. 2003;327(7409):292.

30. Litsios S. The Christian Medical Commission and the development of the World Health Organization's primary health care approach. Am J Public Health. 2004 Nov;94(11):1184–93.

Chapter 6. Early Academic Programs

1. Henderson DA. The eradication of smallpox–an overview of the past, present, and future. Vaccine. 2011;29:D7–9.

2. Ellner P. Smallpox: gone but not forgotten. Infection. 1998;26(5):263–69.

3. Morens DM, Holmes EC, Davis AS, Taubenberger JK. Global rinderpest eradication: lessons learned and why humans should celebrate too. J Infect Dis. 2011;204(4):502–5.

4. Fee E. Disease and discovery: a history of the Johns Hopkins School of Hygiene and Public Health, 1916–1939. Baltimore, MD: Johns Hopkins University Press; 2016.

5. Choi BC. The past, present, and future of public health surveillance. Scientifica. 2012 Oct.

6. Health BUSoP. A brief history of public health: public health in the United States. https://sphweb.bumc.bu.edu/otlt/mph-modules/ph/publichealthhistory/publichealthhistory8.html. Published 2015. Updated Oct 1, 2015. Accessed March 17, 2021.

7. Committee for the Study of the Future of Public Health IoM. The future of public health. Washington DC: National Academies Press; 1988.

8. Etheridge EW. Sentinel for health: a history of the Centers for Disease Control. Berkeley: Univ of California Press; 1992.

9. Thomas KK. Cultivating hygiene as a science: the Welch-Rose Report's influence at Johns Hopkins and beyond. Am J Epidemiol. 2016;183(5):345–54.

10. Rockefeller Foundation. Public health at Johns Hopkins. Digital History Website. https://rockfound.rockarch.org/public-health-at -johns-hopkins. Published N.D. Accessed November 12, 2020.

11. McCollum EV, Davis M. The necessity of certain lipins in the diet during growth. J Biol Chem. 1913;15(1):167–75.

12. Rosenfeld L. Vitamine—vitamin. The early years of discovery. Clin Chem. 1997;43(4):680–85.

13. Sommer A. The Johns Hopkins Bloomberg School of Public Health: a brief history of a century of epidemiologic discovery. Am J Epidemiol. 2016;183(5):340–44.

14. Williams D. The London School of Tropical Medicine. BMJ. 1902;II:808.

15. Medicine LSoHaT. Historical timeline. https://www.lshtm.ac.uk /research/research-action/lshtm-120/historical-timeline. Published 2021. Accessed November 20, 2020.

16. Tulchinsky TH. John Snow, cholera, the Broad Street pump; Water-borne diseases then and now. Case Stud Public Health. 2018:77.

17. Cook G. Early history of clinical tropical medicine in London. J R Soc Med. 1990;83(1):38–41.

18. Acheson R, Poole P. The London School of Hygiene and Tropical Medicine: a child of many parents. Med Hist. 1991;35(4):385–408.

19. Baker R, Bayliss R. William John Ritchie Simpson (1855–1931): public health and tropical medicine. Med Hist. 1987;31(4):450–65.

20. Doll R, Hill AB. Smoking and carcinoma of the lung. BMJ. 1950;2(4682):739.

21. Graham W, Brass W, Snow RW. Estimating maternal mortality: the sisterhood method. Stud Fam Plann. 1989 May 1;20(3):125–35.

22. Duffy TP. The Flexner report—100 years later. Yale J Biol Med. 2011;84(3):269.

23. Flexner A. Medical education in the United States and Canada. Science. 1910;32(810):41–50.

24. Steinecke A, Terrell C. Progress for whose future? The impact of the Flexner Report on medical education for racial and ethnic minority physicians in the United States. Acad Med. 2010; 85(2):236–45.

25. Wellman C. The New Orleans School of Tropical Medicine, and Hygiene. Am J Epidemiol. 2012;176(7).

26. Buekens P. From hygiene and tropical medicine to global health. Am J Epidemiol. 2012;176(suppl_7):S1–3.

27. Scott CK. Life is too short: an autobiography. Philadelphia: Lippincott; 1943.

28. Rodriguez A, Vargas AG. Campus maintains connections to legendary capitalist with legacy of colonization. The Tulane Hullabaloo. https://tulanehullabaloo.com/41022/news/zemurray/. Published 2018. Accessed March 5, 2021.

29. Dyer JP. Tulane: the biography of a university, 1834–1965. New York: Harper & Row; 1966.

30. Sullivan LW, Mittman IS. The state of diversity in the health professions a century after Flexner. Acad Med. 2010;85(2):246–53.

Chapter 7. Bilateral Programs

1. Congress.gov. S.1104—113th Congress (2013–2014): Assessing progress in Haiti Act of 2014. 2014 Aug 8. https://www.congress.gov/bill/113th-congress/senate-bill/1104.

2. US Agency for International Development. Earthquake overview | Basic Page | Haiti. 2022 Jul 18. https://www.usaid.gov/haiti/earthquake-overview.

3. UN News. Haiti cholera outbreak "stopped in its tracks." 2020 Jan 24. https://news.un.org/en/story/2020/01/1056021.

4. Melito M. INTERNATIONAL FOOD ASSISTANCE cargo preference increases food aid shipping costs, and benefits are unclear. Highlights of GAO-15–666, a report to congressional requesters. GAO. 2015 Aug. https://www.gao.gov/assets/gao-15-666.pdf.

5. Louis Picard L, Buss T. Fragile balance: re-examining the history of foreign aid, security and diplomacy. West Hartford, CT: Kumarian Press; 2009.

6. Leffler MP. The United States and the strategic dimensions of the Marshall Plan. Dipl Hist. 1988;12(3):277–306. http://www.jstor.org/stable/24911804.

7. US Agency for International Development. USAID history. 2022 Dec 15. https://www.usaid.gov/about-us/usaid-history.

8. Special message to the Congress on foreign aid. 1961 Mar 22. https://www.presidency.ucsb.edu/documents/special-message-the-congress-foreign-aid-1.

9. Leepson M. The heart and mind of USAID's Vietnam mission. Foreign Serv J. 2000 Apr:20-7.

10. Carrier JM, Thomson CAH. Viet Cong motivation and morale: the special case of Chieu Hoi. Memorandum RM-4830-2-ISA/ARPA. 1966 May. https://www.rand.org/content/dam/rand/pubs/research _memoranda/2006/RM4830-2.pdf.

11. Kelle M. Where we were in Vietnam: a comprehensive guide to the firebases, military installations, and naval vessels of the Vietnam War. Central Point (OR): Hellgate Press; 2002.

12. Phillips R. Why Vietnam matters: an eyewitness account of lessons not learned. Annapolis (MD): Naval Institute Press; 2008.

13. Mullaney A, Hassan SA. He led the CIA to Bin Laden—and unwittingly fueled a vaccine backlash. National Geographic. 2015 Feb 27. https://www.nationalgeographic.com/science/article/150227 -polio-pakistan-vaccination-taliban-osama-bin-laden.

14. Bendavid E. Past and future performance: PEPFAR in the landscape of foreign aid for health. Curr HIV/AIDS Rep. 2016 Oct;13(5): 256–62. https://doi.org/10.1007/s11904-016-0326-8.

15. Fidler DP. Fighting the axis of Illness: HIV/AIDS, human rights, and U.S. foreign policy. Harv Hum Rights J. 2004(17):99.

16. Moss K, Kates J. PEPFAR reauthorization: side-by-side of legislation over time. Kaiser Family Foundation. 2022 Aug 18. https:// www.kff.org/global-health-policy/issue-brief/pepfar-reauthorization -side-by-side-of-existing-and-proposed-legislation/.

17. Lo NC, Lowe A, Bendavid E. The impact of PEPFAR abstinence and faithfulness funding upon HIV risk behaviors in Sub-Saharan Africa. Conference on Retroviruses and Opportunistic Infections. 2015 Feb 23–26; Seattle, WA.

18. Masenior NF, Beyrer C. The US anti-prostitution pledge: First Amendment challenges and public health priorities. PLoS Med4 2007 Jul 24;(7):e207. https://doi.org/10.1371/journal.pmed.0040207.

19. Garrett L. The challenge of global health. Foreign Aff. 2007; 86(1):14–38.

20. Nixon SA, Lee K, Bhutta ZA, Blanchard J, Haddad S, Hoffman SJ, Tugwell P, et al. Canada's global health role: supporting equity and global citizenship as a middle power. Lancet 2018 Apr;391(10131) :1736–48. https://doi.org/10.1016/S0140-6736(18)30322-2.

21. Parisi L. Canada's new Feminist International Assistance Policy: business as usual? Foreign Policy Anal. 2020 Apr 1;16(2):163–80. https://doi.org/10.1093/fpa/orz027.

22. Global Affairs Canada. Canada's Feminist International Assistance Policy: #HerVoiceHerChoice." Ottowa, Ontario, Canada: Global Affairs Canada. 2017. https://www.international.gc.ca/world -monde/assets/pdfs/iap2-eng.pdf?_ga=2.209486491.826559497 .1671582007–1696293316.1671582007.

23. Tiessen R. What's new about Canada's Feminist International Assistance Policy: the problem and possibilities of 'more of the same.' School of Public Policy Publications. 2019 Dec;12(44).

24. Global Affairs Canada. Minister Gould announces support for sexual and reproductive health and rights [News release]. 2020 Jun 22. https://www.canada.ca/en/global-affairs/news/2020/06/minister -gould-announces-support-for-sexual-and-reproductive-health-and -rights.html.

25. Rao S, Tiessen R. Whose feminism(s)? Overseas partner organizations' perceptions of Canada's Feminist International Assistance Policy. Intl J. 2020 Sep 1;75(3):349–66. https://doi.org/10.1177/0020702 020960120.

26. Spiegel JM, Huish R. Canadian foreign aid for global health: human security opportunity lost. Can Foreign Policy J. 2009 Jan;15;3:60–84. https://doi.org/10.1080/11926422.2009 .9673492.

27. Chang AY, Cowling K, Micah AE, Chapin A, Chen CS, Ikilezi G, Sadat N, et al. Past, present, and future of global health financing: a review of development assistance, government, out-of-pocket, and other private spending on health for 195 countries, 1995–2050. Lancet. 2019 Jun 1;393(10187):2233–60. https://doi.org/10.1016 /S0140-6736(19)30841-4.

28. George E. The Cuban intervention in Angola, 1965 - 1991: from Che Guevara to Cuito Cuanavale. 1. issued in paperback. Cass Military Studies. London: Routledge; 2012.

29. Londoño E. Cuban doctors revolt: 'You get tired of being a slave.' New York Times. 2017 Sep 29. sec. World. https://www.nytimes .com/2017/09/29/world/americas/brazil-cuban-doctors-revolt .html.

30. Alves L. Cuba's doctors-abroad programme comes under fire. Lancet. 2019 Sep 28:394(10204):1132. https://doi.org/10.1016 /S0140-6736(19)32214-7.

31. Ceaser M. Cuban doctors working abroad defect to the USA. Lancet. 2007 Apr 14;369(9569):1247–48. https://doi.org/10.1016 /S0140-6736(07)60577-7.

32. Irwin R. Sweden's engagement in global health: a historical review. Glob Health. 2019 Nov 26;15(1):79. https://doi.org/10.1186/s12992-019-0499-1.

33. Barboza D. China unveils $586 billion stimulus plan. New York Times. 2008 Nov 10. sec. World. https://www.nytimes.com/2008/11/10/world/asia/10iht-10china.17673270.html.

34. Malik AA, Parks B, Russell B, Lin J, Walsh K, Solomon K, Zhang S, Elston T-B, Goodman S. Banking on the belt and road. Policy Rep. AIDDATA. n.d. https://www.aiddata.org/publications/banking-on-the-belt-and-road.

35. Hu D, Zhu W, Fu Y, Zhang M, Zhao Y, Hanson K, Martinez-Alvarez M, Liu X. Development of village doctors in China: financial compensation and health system support. Int J Equity Health. 2017 Jul 1:16(1):9. https://doi.org/10.1186/s12939-016-0505-7.

36. Li LA. The edge of expertise: representing barefoot doctors in cultural revolution China. Endeavour. 2015 Sep-Dec:39(3–4):160–67. https://doi.org/10.1016/j.endeavour.2015.05.007.

37. Gauttam P, Singh B, Kaur J. COVID-19 and Chinese global health diplomacy: geopolitical opportunity for China's hegemony? Millenn Asia. 2020 Dec 1:11(3):318–40. https://doi.org/10.1177/09763996 20959771.

38. Wang J, Xu C, Wong YK, Li Y, Liao F, Jiang T, Tu Y. Artemisinin, the magic drug discovered from traditional Chinese medicine. Engineering. 2019 Feb:5(1):32–39. https://doi.org/10.1016/j.eng .2018.11.011.

39. Krishna S, Bustamante L, Haynes RK, Staines HM. Artemisinins: their growing importance in medicine. Trends Pharmacol Sci. 2008 Oct:29(10):520–27. https://doi.org/10.1016/j.tips.2008.07.004.

40. Data: Chinese investment in Africa. China Africa Research Initiative, Johns Hopkins School of Advanced International Studies. http://www.sais-cari.org/chinese-investment-in-africa. Accessed December 20, 2022.

41. Olander E. China sends medical teams to Africa as part of new, stepped-up aid push. The China Global South Project. Accessed December 20, 2022. https://chinaglobalsouth.com/analysis/china-sends-medical-teams-to-africa-as-part-of-new-stepped-up-aid-push/.

42. Grépin KA, Fan VY, Shen GC, Chen L. China's role as a global health donor in Africa: what can we learn from studying under

reported resource flows? Global Health. 2014 Dec 30:84. https://doi
.org/10.1186/s12992-014-0084-6.

43. News Agency of Nigeria. Coronavirus: NUJ begs FG to avoid
Chinese medical team. Pulse Nigeria. 2020 Apr 4. https://www.pulse
.ng/news/local/coronavirus-nuj-begs-fg-to-avoid-chinese-medical
-team/2kbrt9s.

44. Daly G, Kaufman J, Lin S, Gao L, Reyes M, Matemu S, El-Sadr W.
Challenges and opportunities in China's health aid to Africa: findings
from qualitative interviews in Tanzania and Malawi. Global Health.
2020 Dec:16(71). https://doi.org/10.1186/s12992-020-00577-0.

Chapter 8. Multilateral Organizations

1. Wee Sui-Lee, McNeil DG, Jr, Hernández JC. W.H.O. declares global
emergency as Wuhan Coronavirus spreads. New York Times. 2020
Jan 30;Sect Health. https://www.nytimes.com/2020/01/30/health
/coronavirus-world-health-organization.html.

2. Qin A, Li C. China pushes for quiet burials as Coronavirus death
toll is questioned. New York Times. 2020 Apr 3;Sect. World.
https://www.nytimes.com/2020/04/03/world/asia/coronavirus
-china-grief-deaths.html.

3. Salaam-Blyther T, Blanchfield L, Weed MC, Gill CR. U.S. with-
drawal from the World Health Organization: process and implications. CRS Report. Congressional Research Service. 2020 Oct 21.
https://crsreports.congress.gov/product/pdf/R/R46575.

4. Biden JR, Jr. Letter to His Excellency António Guterres. 2021 Jan
21. https://www.whitehouse.gov/briefing-room/statements-releases
/2021/01/20/letter-his-excellency-antonio-guterres/.

5. Constitution of the World Health Organization. Adopted by the
International Health Conference; 1946 Jul 22. https://apps.who.int
/gb/bd/PDF/bd47/EN/constitution-en.pdf.

6. Charles J. Origins, history, and achievements of the World Health
Organization. Br Med J. 1968 May 4;2(5600): 293–96. https://doi
.org/10.1136/bmj.2.5600.293.

7. Report of the International Conference on Primary Health Care.
Alma-Ata, USSR: World Health Organization and United Nations
Children's Fund; 1978 Sep 6. https://www.unicef.org/documents
/alma-ata-primary-healthcare-conference.

8. World Health Organization. China's village doctors take great
strides. Bull World Health Organ. 2008 Dec;86(12): 909–88.

9. Rifkin SB. Alma Ata after 40 Years: primary health care and health for all—from consensus to complexity. BMJ Glob Health. 2018 Dec 20;3(Suppl):e001188. https://doi.org/10.1136/bmjgh-2018-001188.

10. World Health Organization. Smallpox: historical significance. 2007 Sep 21. Factsheet. https://web.archive.org/web/20070921235036/http://www.who.int/mediacentre/factsheets/smallpox/en/.

11. WHO Framework Convention on Tobacco Control and World Health Organization. WHO Framework Convention on Tobacco Control. 2003:36 Convention-cadre de l' OMS pour la lutte antitabac.

12. Puska P, Daube M. Impact assessment of the WHO Framework Convention on Tobacco Control: introduction, general findings and discussion. Tobacco Control. 2019 Jun;28(Suppl 2): s81–s83. https://doi.org/10.1136/tobaccocontrol-2018-054429.

13. Gravely S, Giovino GA, Craig L, Commar A, D'Espaignet ET, Schotte K, GT Fong. Implementation of key demand-reduction measures of the WHO Framework Convention on Tobacco Control and change in smoking prevalence in 126 countries: an association study. Lancet Public Health. 2017 Apr;2(4): e166–74. https://doi.org/10.1016/S2468-2667(17)30045-2.

14. Zhou SY, Liberman JD, Ricafort E. The impact of the WHO Framework Convention on Tobacco Control in defending legal challenges to tobacco control measures. Tobacco Control. 2019 Jun 1;28(Suppl 2):s113. https://doi.org/10.1136/tobaccocontrol-2018-054329.

15. World Health Organization. Thirteenth General Programme of Work 2019–2023. 2018 May 25. https://www.who.int/about/general-programme-of-work/thirteenth.

16. World Health Organization. Proposed programme budget 2022–2023. Geneva: WHO; 2021. https://apps.who.int/iris/bitstream/handle/10665/346071/9789240036109-eng.pdf.

17. Centers for Disease Control and Prevention. FY 2023 CDC budget detail. 2022 Mar 28. https://www.cdc.gov/budget/documents/fy2023/FY-2023-CDC-Budget-Detail.pdf.

18. The U.S. Government and the World Health Organization. KFF (blog). 2022. https://www.kff.org/coronavirus-covid-19/fact-sheet/the-u-s-government-and-the-world-health-organization/.

19. World Health Organization. The WHO Programme Budget Portal, 2020–21. https://open.who.int/2020-21/home.

20. World Health Organization. Contingency Fund for Emergencies (CFE). https://www.who.int/emergencies/funding/contingency-fund-for-emergencies. Accessed January 9, 2023.

21. Health conditions in the occupied Palestinian Territory, including East Jerusalem, and in the occupied Syrian Golan. Geneva: Seventy-Fourth World Health Assembly. n.d.
22. UN Watch. WHO's 2022 Assembly singles out Israel as violator of health rights. 2022 May 25. https://unwatch.org/who-2022-assembly-singles-out-israel-violator-health-rights/.
23. Wong T. Why Taiwan has become a problem for WHO. BBC News. 2020 Mar 30.Sect. Asia. https://www.bbc.com/news/world-asia-52088167.
24. Chien E. Beyond SARS: give Taiwan WHO status. International Herald Tribune. New York Times. 2003 May 16;Sect. Opinion. https://www.nytimes.com/2003/05/16/opinion/IHT-beyond-sars-give-taiwan-who-status.html.
25. Cyranoski D. Taiwan left isolated in fight against SARS. Nature. 2003 Apr;422, 652. https://doi.org/10.1038/422652a.
26. Buranyi S. The WHO v Coronavirus: why it can't handle the pandemic. The Guardian 2020 Apr 10;Sect. News. https://www.theguardian.com/news/2020/apr/10/world-health-organization-who-v-coronavirus-why-it-cant-handle-pandemic.
27. Sridhar D, Winters J, Strong E. World Bank's financing, priorities, and lending structures for global health. BMJ. 2017 Aug 31;j3339. https://doi.org/10.1136/bmj.j3339.
28. Moss K. Donor funding for the global novel Coronavirus response. Kaiser Family Foundation. 2020 Apr 23. https://www.kff.org/coronavirus-covid-19/issue-brief/donor-funding-for-the-global-novel-coronavirus-response/.
29. Elmendorf AE. Global health: then and now. UN Chronicle (blog). United Nations. https://www.un.org/en/chronicle/article/global-health-then-and-now. Accessed January 9, 2023.
30. World Bank. Digitized records of the World Bank's first loan. Text/HTML. https://www.worldbank.org/en/archive/history/exhibits/Digitized-Records-World-Bank-First-Loan. Accessed January 9, 2023.
31. Obama names surprise World Bank candidate Jim Yong Kim. BBC News. 2012 Mar 23;Sect. Business. https://www.bbc.com/news/business-17481973.
32. Packard RM. A history of global health: interventions into the lives of other peoples. Baltimore, MD: Johns Hopkins University Press; 2016.
33. Kim JY. World Bank group president Jim Yong Kim's speech at World Health Assembly: poverty, health and the human future.

Presented at the World Health Assembly; 2013 May 21; Geneva. https://www.worldbank.org/en/news/speech/2013/05/21/world -bank-group-president-jim-yong-kim-speech-at-world-health -assembly.

34. Clinton C, Sridhar DL. Governing global health: who runs the world and why? New York: Oxford University Press; 2017.

35. World Bank. Robert S. McNamara. https://www.worldbank.org/en /archive/history/past-presidents/robert-strange-mcnamara.

36. Lelyveld J. McNamara's style at the World Bank. New York Times. 1975 Nov 30.

37. World Bank. The World Bank in United States. https://www.world bank.org/en/country/unitedstates/overview. Accessed January 9, 2023.

38. Woods N. The United States and the international financial institutions: power and influence within the World Bank and the IMF. In: Foot R, MacFarlane SN, Mastanduno M, editors. US hegemony and international organizations. Oxford: Oxford University Press; 2003:92–114. https://doi.org/10.1093/0199261431.003 .0005.

39. Secretary-general proposes global fund for fight against HIV/AIDS and other infectious diseases at African leaders summit. UN Press. 2001 Apr 26. https://press.un.org/en/2001/SGSM7779R1.doc.htm.

40. Global AIDS fund should be up and running by year's end, Annan says. UN News. 2001 Jun 27. https://news.un.org/en/story/2001/06 /4102.

41. The Global Fund. Results Report 2021. https://archive.the globalfund.org/media/11304/archive_2021-results-report_report _en.pdf.

42. The Global Fund. Global Fund statement on abuse of funds in some countries. 2011 Jan 24. https://www.theglobalfund.org/en/news /2011/2011-01-24-gobal-fund-statement-on-abuse-of-funds-in-some -countries/.

43. The Global Fund. Nhin Kpă from La Rsươm, Viet Nam. 2022 Feb 11. https://www.theglobalfund.org/en/stories/2022/2022-02-11-nhin -kpa-from-la-rsuom-viet-nam/.

44. The Global Fund. Zambia: solar power fuels better health. 2022 Feb 17. https://www.theglobalfund.org/en/stories/2022/2022-02-17 -zambia-solar-power-fuels-better-health/.

45. Kaiser Family Foundation. The U.S. & the Global Fund to fight AIDS, tuberculosis and malaria. 2022 Sep 9, 2022. https://www.kff

.org/global-health-policy/fact-sheet/the-u-s-the-global-fund-to-fight
-aids-tuberculosis-and-malaria/.

46. Sidibe M, Ramiah I, Buse K. The Global Fund at five: what next for universal access for HIV/AIDS, TB and malaria? J R Soc Med. 2006 Oct;99(10):497–500. https://doi.org/10.1177/01410768060 9901010.

47. Hanefeld J. The Global Fund to fight AIDS, tuberculosis and malaria: 10 years on. J Clin Med. 2014 Feb;14(1):54–57. https://doi .org/10.7861/clinmedicine.14-1-54.

48. Hanefeld J. The impact of global health initiatives at national and sub-national level—a policy analysis of their role in implementation processes of antiretroviral treatment (ART) roll-out in Zambia and South Africa. AIDS Care. 2010;22(Suppl 1):93–102. https://doi.org /10.1080/09540121003759919.

49. Hanefeld J, Musheke M. What impact do Global Health Initiatives have on human resources for antiretroviral treatment roll-out? A qualitative policy analysis of implementation processes in Zambia. Hum Resour Health. 2009 Feb 10:7(8). https://doi.org/10.1186 /1478-4491-7-8.

50. Fan VY, Duran D, Silverman R, Glassman A. Performance-based financing at the Global Fund to Fight AIDS, Tuberculosis and Malaria: an analysis of grant ratings and funding, 2003–12. Lancet Global Health. 2013 Sep;1(3):e161–68. https://doi.org/10.1016 /S2214-109X(13)70017-2.

51. The Global Fund. (RED). https://www.theglobalfund.org/en/private -ngo-partners/resource-mobilization/red/.

52. Food and Drug Administration. COVID-19 tests and collection kits authorized by the FDA: infographic. 2021 Oct 18. https:// clpmag.com/disease-states/infectious-diseases/covid-19/fda -publishes-infographic-on-authorized-covid-19-tests-and-collection -kits/.

53. World Health Organization. The ACT-Accelerator frequently asked questions. https://www.who.int/initiatives/act-accelerator/faq. Accessed August 5, 2022.

54. Le TT, Cramer JP, Chen R, Mayhew S. Evolution of the COVID-19 vaccine development landscape. Nat Rev Drug Discov. 2020 Oct;19(10):667–68. https://doi.org/10.1038/d41573-020-00151-8.

55. World Health Organization. What is the Access to COVID-19 Tools (ACT) Accelerator, how is it structured and how does it work? 2021 Apr 21. https://www.who.int/publications/m/item/what-is-the-access

-to-covid-19-tools-(act)-accelerator-how-is-it-structured-and-how
-does-it-work.

56. Mullard A. How COVID vaccines are being divvied up around the world. Nature. 2020 Nov 30; d41586-020-03370–76. https://doi.org/10.1038/d41586-020-03370-6.

57. Government of Canada. Canada's COVID-19 vaccine supply and donation strategy. 2022 May 16. https://www.canada.ca/en/public-health/services/diseases/coronavirus-disease-covid-19/vaccines/supply-donation.html.

58. UN News. WHO chief warns against 'catastrophic moral failure' in COVID-19 vaccine access. 2021 Jan 18. https://news.un.org/en/story/2021/01/1082362.

59. Hinnant L, Cheng M. Stalled at first jab: vaccine shortages hit poor countries. AP News. 2021 Apr 10. https://apnews.com/article/middle-east-coronavirus-pandemic-united-nations-b52bf58e35031e71a5ff85f7a59244f8.

60. Cohen J. 'I'm still feeling that we're failing': exasperated WHO leader speaks out about vaccine inequity. Science. 2021 Jun 18. https://www.science.org/content/article/i-m-still-feeling-we-re-failing-exasperated-who-leader-speaks-out-about-vaccine.

61. Paun C. Gavi on the defensive over vaccine-equity effort. POLITICO. 2021 Aug 5. https://www.politico.com/newsletters/global-pulse/2021/08/05/gavi-on-the-defensive-over-vaccine-equity-effort-493855.

62. Africa CDC. COVID-19 vaccination—Africa CDC. https://africacdc.org/covid-19-vaccination/. Accessed August 5, 2022.

63. Black M. The Children and the Nations: The Story of UNICEF. 1986. United Nations Children's Fund.

64. The National Archives. "Iron curtain" speech [Text]. https://www.nationalarchives.gov.uk/education/resources/cold-war-on-file/iron-curtain-speech/. Accessed April 10, 2021.

65. UNICEF. UNICEF—UNICEF History—Milestones: 1946–1956. http://www.cf-hst.net/unicef-temp/cf-hst%20redesign/milestones%2046-56.htm. Accessed December 6, 2020.

66. Adamson P, Jolly R, UNICEF. Jim Grant: UNICEF Visionary. 2001. UNICEF Innocenti Research Centre.

Chapter 9. The Rise of NGOs

1. Campbell W. The history of CARE: a personal account. Westport, CN: Praeger, 1990.

2. Farmer P. Reimagining global health: an introduction. 1st ed. Vol. 26. Berkeley: University of California Press; 2013.

3. IRIN News. The refugee camp that became a city. United Nations Africa Renewal, n.d. https://www.un.org/africarenewal/news/refugee -camp-became-city.

4. Moss K, Kates J. The role of NGOs in the U.S. global health response. Kaiser Family Foundation Global Health Policy. 2015 Jul 21. https://www.kff.org/global-health-policy/issue-brief/data-note -role-of-ngos-u-s-global-health-response/.

5. Werker E, Ahmed FZ. What do nongovernmental organizations do? JEP. 2008 Spring;22(2):73–92.

6. Hall-Jones P. The rise and rise of NGOs. Global Policy Forum Public Services International. 2006 May. https://archive.globalpolicy .org/component/content/article/176-general/31937.html.

7. Gellert G. Non-governmental organizations in international health: past successes, future challenges. Int J Health Plan Manag. 1996; 11(1):19–31.

8. Yaziji M, Doh J. NGOs and corporations: conflict and collabora- tion. Cambridge: Cambridge University Press; 2009.

9. Iriye A. A century of NGOs. Dipl Hist. 1999 Summer;23(3): 421–35.

10. Martens K. NGOs and the United Nations, professionalization and adaptation. Basingstoke: Palgrave MacMillan; 2006.

11. Forsythe D. The humanitarians. International Committee of the Red Cross: Cambridge (UK): Cambridge University Press; 2005.

12. Forsythe D, Rieffer-Flanagan B. A neutral humanitarian actor. Inter- national Committee of the Red Cross. Milton Park (UK): Routledge; 2007.

13. Ryfman P. Non-governmental organizations: an indispensable player of humanitarian aid. Int Rev Red Cross. 2005;89(865): 21–46.

14. Gaist PA. Igniting the power of community: the role of CBOs and NGOs in global public health. New York (NY): Springer; 2010.

15. Knudsen R. USAID history. USAID who we are (n.d.). https://www .usaid.gov/who-we-are/usaid-history.

16. Chacho TM. The U.S. military-NGO relationship in post-WWII Germany. Combat Studies Institute Symposium United States Military Academy; 2008 Sep.

17. Chimini BS. The meaning of words and the role of UNHCR in voluntary repatriation. Int J Refug Law. 1993 Jan:5(3):442–60.

18. Berthiaume C. Refugees Magazine - Issue 97 (NGOs and UNHCR) - NGOs: our right arm. UNHCR. 1994 Sep. https://www.unhcr.org /en-us/publications/refugeemag/3b53fd8b4/refugees-magazine-issue -97-ngos-unhcr-ngos-right-arm.html.

19. Lowe K. NGOs: A New History of Transnational Civil Society by Thomas Davies, and: Shaping the Transnational Sphere: Experts, Networks and Issues from the 1840s to the 1930s [Review]. In: Rodogno D, Struck B, Vogel J, editors. J World Hist. 2016;26(4): 893–97.

20. Smillie I. NGOs and development assistance: a change in mind-set? In: Weiss TG, editor. Beyond UN subcontracting. International Political Economy Series. London: Palgrave Macmillan; 1998. https://doi.org/10.1007/978-1-349-26263-2_9.

21. Makoba JW. Non governmental organizations and Third World development: an alternative approach to development. J Third World Stud. 2002 Spring;19(1):53–63.

22. Shuller M, Farmer P. Killing with kindness: Haiti, international aid, and NGOs. Piscataway, NJ: Rutgers University Press; 2012.

23. Pfeiffer J. International NGOs and primary health care in Mozambique: the need for a new model of collaboration. SSM. 1982;56(2): 725–38.

24. Lasse H, Moses D. The Nigeria-Biafra War: postcolonial conflict and the question of genocide. J Genocide Res. 2014;16(2): 169–203.

25. Desgrandchamps M-L, Heerten L, Omaka AO, O'Sullivan K, Bertrand T. Biafra, humanitarian intervention and history. J Humanitarian Affairs. 2020 Dec;2(2):68–78.

26. Shampo MA, Kyle RA. Bernard Kouchner—founder of Doctors Without Borders. Mayo Clinic Proc. 2011;86(1). https://doi.org/10 .4065/mcp.2010.0796.

27. Drain P, Huffman S, Pirtle S, Chan K. Caring for the world a guidebook to global health opportunities. Toronto: University of Toronto Press; 2008.

28. Mercer A, Liskin L, Scott S. The role of non-governmental organizations in the global response to AIDS. AIDS Care. 1991;3(3): 265–70.

29. Alizadeh M, Abbasi M, Bashirivand N, Karimi SE. Nongovernmental organizations and social aspects of COVID-19 pandemic: a successful experience in health policy. Med J Islam Repub Iran. 2020;34:170. https://doi.org/10.47176/mjiri.34.170.

30. Parkhurst JO. The Ugandan success story? evidence and claims of HIV-1 prevention. Lancet. 2002;360(9326):78–80.

31. Kiweewa JM. Uganda's HIV/AIDS success story: reviewing the evidence. Journal of Development and Social Transformation. 2008 Nov;5.

32. Missoni E, Alesani D. Management of international institutions and NGOs. London: Routledge; 2013.

33. Muriisa R. The AIDS pandemic in Uganda: social capital and the role of NGOs in alleviating the impact of HIV/AIDS [dissertation]. The University of Bergen; 2007.

34. Kaleeba N, Kalibala S, Kaseje M, Ssebbanja P, Anderson S, van Praag E, Tembo G, Katabira E. Participatory evaluation of counselling, medical and social services of The AIDS Support Organization (TASO) in Uganda. AIDS Care. 1997;9(1):13–26.

35. Green EC, Halperin D, Nantulya V, Hogle JA. Uganda's HIV prevention success: the role of sexual behavior change and the national response. AIDS Behav. 2006 Jul;10(4):335–46.

36. Karpf T. Faith and health: past and present of relations between faith communities and the World Health Organization. Christian Journal for Global Health. 2014;1(1). https://doi.org/10.15566/cjgh.viii.21.

37. Cooper AF, Kirton J, Schrechker T, editors. Governing global health: challenge, response, innovation. Routledge. Taylor and Francis Group; 2007.

38. Matthews D. WTO decision on implementation of paragraph 6 of the DOHA Declaration on the TRIPS Agreement and public health: a solution to the access to essential medicines problem? J Int Econ Law. 2004 Mar 1;7(1):73–107. https://doi.org/10.1093/jiel/7.1.73.

39. World Trade Organization. Developing country group's paper. TRIPS: council discussion on access to medicines trips and public health (2001). https://www.wto.org/english/tratop_e/trips_e/paper_develop_w296_e.htm.

40. World Trade Organization. Re-thinking trips in the WTO: NGOs demand review and reform of TRIPS at Doha Ministerial Conference. La Via Campesina; 2001 Oct 31. https://viacampesina.org/en/re-thinking-trips-in-the-wto-ngos-demand-review-and-reform-of-trips-at-doha-ministerial-conference/.

41. CARE. White House taps CARE to help train Peace Corps volunteers under Let Girls Learn Initiative. CISION PR Newswire. 2015 Mar 3. https://www.prnewswire.com/news-releases/white-house

-taps-care-to-help-train-peace-corps-volunteers-under-let-girls-learn
-initiative-300043960.html.

42. Martins S, Langehaug E, Moeller M-L, Keuhas B. First consolidated CARE International (CI) gender report on the implementation of the CARE gender policy. Report synthesis. 2011. CARE
International Gender Network; 2011.

43. Welankiwar R. CARE CEO Helene Gayle on shaking up a vener-
able organization. Harvard Business Review. 2009. Apr. https://hbr
.org/2009/04/care-ceo-helene-gayle-on-shaking-up-a-venerable
-organization.

44. Palazuelos D, Farmer PE, Mukherjee J. Community health and equity
of outcomes: the Partners In Health experience. Lancet Global Health.
2018;6(5):e491–93.

45. Moschella MC. Accompaniment, abundance, and joy: Paul Farmer
and Partners. In Health. In: Caring for joy: narrative, theology, and
practice. Leiden (NL): Brill; 2016:190–215. https://doi.org/10.1163
/9789004325005_009.

46. Hamblin J. The moral medical mission: Partners In Health,
25 years on. Atlantic, 2012. https://www.theatlantic.com/health
/archive/2012/10/the-moral-medical-mission-partners-in-health-25
-years-on/262974/.

47. Kidder T. Recovering from disaster—Partners In Health and the
Haitian earthquake. N Engl J Med. 2010 Mar 4;362:769–72.
https://doi.org/10.1056/NEJMp1001705.

48. Smillie I. Freedom from want: the remarkable success story of
BRAC, the Global grassroots organization that's winning the fight
against poverty. Boulder: Lynne Rienner Publishers; 2009.

49. French M, Ahmed S. Scaling up: the BRAC experience. BRAC
University Journal. 2006;3(2):35–40.

50. Hadi A. Promoting health knowledge through micro-credit
programmes: experience of BRAC in Bangladesh. Health Promot
Int. 2001;16(3):219–27.

51. Paul S. Knowledge and attitude of key community members towards
tuberculosis: mixed method study from BRAC TB control areas in
Bangladesh. BMC Public Health. 2015;15(1):52.

52. Raza WA, Das NC, Misha FA. Can ultra-poverty be sustainably
improved? Evidence from BRAC in Bangladesh. J Dev Effect.
2012;4(2):257–76.

53. Chowdhury AMR, Jenkins A, Nandita MM. Measuring the effects
of interventions in BRAC, and how this has driven 'development.'

J Dev Effect. 2014;6(4):407–24. https://doi.org/10.1080/19439342 .2014.966452.

54. Halder S, Mosely P. Working with the ultra-poor: learning from BRAC experiences. J Def Effect. 2004;16(3):387–406.

55. The Economist 2010. https://www.economist.com/business/2010/02 /18/brac-in-business.

56. Mommers C, van Wessel M. Structures, values, and interaction in field-level partnerships: the case of UNHCR and NGOs. Development in Practice. 2009;19(2):160–72. https://doi.org/10.1080 /09614520802689428.

57. Glasman J. Seeing like a refugee agency: a short history of UNHCR classifications in Central Africa (1961–2015). J Refug Stud. 2017; 30(2):337–62.

58. Doocy S, Tappis H, Haskew C, Wilkinson C. Performance of UNHCR nutrition programs in post-emergency refugee camps. Conflict and Health. 2011;5(1):23.

59. Cannon B, Fujibayashi H. Security, structural factors and sovereignty: analysing reactions to Kenya's decision to close the Dadaab refugee camp complex. African Security Review. 2018 Jan 2;27(1): 20–41.

60. Hujale M. Returning to Dadaab. The New Humanitarian. 2019. https://www.thenewhumanitarian.org/opinion/first-person/2019/01 /24/Kenya-dadaab-camp-returning.

61. World Vision Kenya Joint statement. Closure of Dadaab and Kakuma Refugee Camps. 2016. https://www.wvi.org/pressrelease /closure-dadaab-and-kakuma-refugee-camps.

62. d'Orsi C. A look at global changes in refugee policies through the lens of Dadaab. The Conversation. 2020 Jun 18. https://theconver sation.com/a-look-at-global-changes-in-refugee-policies-through-the -lens-of-dadaab-140955.

63. Mahmood J. The role of non-governmental organizations in pandemic preparedness. Pandemic Preparedness in Asia. 2009: 113–16.

64. Shin Y, Yeo J, Jung K. The effectiveness of international non-governmental organizations' response operations during public health emergency: lessons learned from the 2014 Ebola outbreak in Sierra Leone. Int J Environ Res Public Health. 2018; Apr 1;15(4):650. https://www.semanticscholar.org/paper/The-Effective ness-of-International-Non-Governmental-Shin-Yeo/0566aa707f3b 1ad42785c81a90020abd489cf158.

65. Mohseni M, Azami-Aghdash S, Isfahani HM, Moosavi A, Fardid M. Role of nongovernmental organizations in controlling COVID-19. Dis Med Public Health Prep. 2022 Oct;16(5):1705.

66. Cai Q, Okada A, Jeong BG, Kim S-J. Civil society responses to the COVID-19 pandemic: a comparative study of China, Japan, and South Korea. China Review. 2021 Feb;21(1):107–37.

67. Gideon J, Porter F. Challenging gendered inequalities in global health: dilemmas for NGOs: debate: challenging gendered inequalities in global health. Development and Change. 2016;47(4): 782–97.

68. Appe S, Barragán D. Universities, NGOs, and civil society sustainability: preliminary lessons from Ecuador. Dev Pract Development. 2017;27(4):472–86. https://doi.org/10.1080/09614524.2017 .1303035.

Chapter 10. Hybrid Organizations

1. Foege WF. The Task Force for Child Survival: secrets of successful coalitions. Baltimore, MD: Johns Hopkins University Press; 2018.

Chapter 11. Early Philanthropy and the Rockefeller Foundation

1. Shubinski B. Evolution of a foundation: an institutional history of the Rockefeller Foundation. Rockefeller Archive Center Global Engagement. Issues in Philanthropy. 2022 Jan 12. https://resource .rockarch.org/story/rockefeller-foundation-history-origins-to-2013/.

2. Council on Foundations. Philanthropy. Glossary of philanthropic terms. n.d. https://cof.org/content/glossary-philanthropic-terms.

3. Wimpee R, Shubinski B. Timeline: American foundations and the history of public health. Rockefeller Archive Center. Issues in Philanthropy. 2011 Dec 11. https://resource.rockarch.org/story /timeline-american-foundations-and-the-history-of-public-health/.

4. Staff. A brief history of billionaire philanthropists and the people who hate them. The Week. 2016 Jan 9. https://theweek.com/articles /597963/brief-history-billionaire-philanthropists-people-who-hate.

5. Rogers D, Keenan T. The role of foundations in American society. Health Aff. 1990;9(4 Winter). https://www.healthaffairs.org/doi/full /10.1377/hlthaff.9.4.186.

6. Karl BD, Katz SN. The American private philanthropic foundation and the public sphere 1890–1930. Minerva. 1981;19(2):236–70. http://www.jstor.org/stable/41820456.

7. Shubinski B, Iacobelli T. Public health: how the fight against hookworm helped build a system. Rockefeller Archive Center Medicine & Public Health. 2020 Apr 23. https://resource.rockarch.org/story/public-health-how-the-fight-against-hookworm-helped-build-a-system/.

8. Farley J. To cast out disease: a history of the International Health Division of Rockefeller Foundation (1913–1951). Cary: Oxford University Press; 2003.

9. Birn A-E, Fee E. The Rockefeller Foundation and the international health agenda. Lancet (Br ed.). 2013;381(9878):1618–19.

10. Andrew Carnegie: The Gospel of wealth. National Center for Family Philanthropy Knowledge Center. 2022 Oct 22. https://www.ncfp.org/knowledge/andrew-carnegie-the-gospel-of-wealth/.

11. PBS. Frederick T. Gates. American Experience. (n.d.). https://www.pbs.org/wgbh/americanexperience/features/rockefellers-gates/.

12. Birn A-E. Philanthrocapitalism, past and present: the Rockefeller Foundation, the Gates Foundation, and the setting(s) of the international/global health agenda. Hypothesis. 2014;12(1). https://archive.wphna.org/wp-content/uploads/2015/04/2014-11-Hypothesis-Anne-Emanuelle-Birn-Rockefeller-and-Gates1.pdf.

13. Our history. The Rockefeller University, n.d. https://www.rockefeller.edu/about/history/.

14. Snyder M. Sour milk: preventing infant mortality with public health. Rockefeller Archive Center. Medicine & Public Health. 2020 May 6. https://resource.rockarch.org/story/sour-milk-preventing-infant-mortality-with-public-health-rockefeller-institute-food-safety-study/.

15. Brown ER. Public health in imperialism: early Rockefeller programs at home and abroad. Am J Public Health. 1971;66(9):897–903.

16. Goldberg B. The long road to the yellow fever vaccine. Rockefeller Archive Center Medicine & Public Health. 2019 Nov 2. https://resource.rockarch.org/story/the-long-road-to-the-yellow-fever-vaccine/.

17. Youde J. The Rockefeller and Gates Foundations in global health governance. Glob Soc. 2013;27(2):139–58.

18. Packard R. A history of global health: interventions into the lives of other peoples. Baltimore, MD: John Hopkins University Press; 2016.

19. Downs W. The Rockefeller Foundation virus program: 1951–1971 with update to 1981. Annu Rev Med. 1982;33:1–30. https://doi.org/10.1146/annurev.me.33.020182.000245.

20. Weindling P. Philanthropy and world health: the Rockefeller Foundation and the League of Nations Health Organisation. Minerva. 1997:35(3):269–81.
21. Fosdick R. The story of the Rockefeller Foundation. New York: Harper & Brothers; 1952:279–99.
22. Schambra WA. Philanthropy's original sin. The New Atlantis. 2013 Summer. https://www.thenewatlantis.com/publications/philanthropys -original-sin.

Chapter 12. The New Philanthropy

1. Moran M, Stevenson M. Illumination and innovation: what philanthropic foundations bring to global health governance. Glob Soc. (n.d.):27(2):117–37. https://doi.org/10.1080/13600826.2012.762343.
2. Bartlett K. The health of nations: the campaign to end polio and eradicate epidemic diseases. London: OneWorld Publications; 2017.
3. Youde J. Private actors, global health and learning the lessons of history. Med Confl Surv. 2016;32(3):203–20. https://doi.org/10 .1080/13623699.2016.1249526.
4. Falcão M, Odeh M, Giugliani S. Global health watch 5: an alternative world health report. Saúde Em Debate. 2020;1(44).
5. Dobrzynski JH. Philanthropy now: diversity and creativity for changing times. Pundicity Carnegie Reporter. 2007 Spring. http:// www.judithdobrzynski.com/3011/philanthropy-now.
6. Stevenson M, Youde J. Public-private partnering as a modus operandi: explaining the Gates Foundation's approach to global health governance. Glob Public Health. 2021;16(3):401–14.
7. Birn A-E. Philanthrocapitalism, past and present: the Rockefeller Foundation, the Gates Foundation, and the setting(s) of the international/global health agenda. Hypothesis 12;2014:12(1). https://www .semanticscholar.org/paper/Philanthrocapitalism,-past-and-present: -The-the-and-Birn/181d48165f9130358d11580513b2eb7891e978da.
8. Youde J. The Rockefeller and Gates Foundations in global health governance. Glob Soc. 2013;27(2):139–58. https://doi.org/10.1080 /13600826.2012.762341.
9. Butler CD. Philanthrocapitalism: promoting global health but failing planetary health. Challenges. 2019;10(24). https://doi.org/10.3390 /challe10010024.
10. Singer P. What should a billionaire give—and what should you? New York Times Magazine. 2006. https://www.nytimes.com/2006 /12/17/magazine/17charity.t.html.

11. Clarke LC. Responsibility of hybrid public-private bodies under international law: a case study of global health public-private partnerships [dissertation]. Amsterdam: University of Amsterdam; 2012.

12. Packard R. A history of global health: interventions into the lives of other peoples. Baltimore, MD: John Hopkins University Press; 2016.

13. Missoni E, Alesani D. Management of international institutions and NGOs. London: Routledge Taylor and Francis Group; 2013.

14. Glassman A, Temin M. Millions saved: new cases of proven success in global health. Washington DC: Brookings Institution Press; 2016.

15. Gates M. The moment of lift: how empowering women changes the world. New York: Flatiron Books; 2019.

16. Cohen J. Gates Foundation rearranges public health universe. Am Assoc Adv Sci. 2002;295(5562):2000.

17. Fejerskov AM. From unconventional to ordinary? The Bill and Melinda Gates Foundation and the homogenizing effects of international development cooperation. J Int Dev. 2015;27(7):1098–112.

18. Bishop M, Green M. Philanthrocapitalism: how giving can save the world. London: Bloomsbury Publishing; 2008.

19. Doughton S. After 10 years, few payoffs from Bill Gates' "Grand Challenges." Seattle Times; 2014. https://www.seattletimes.com/seattle-news/after-10-years-few-payoffs-from-gatesrsquo-lsquogrand-challengesrsquo/.

20. What has the Gates Foundation done for global health? Lancet [editorial]. 2003 May 9;373(9675):1577.

21. Rogers P. The Mercury News Health (2020). https://www.mercurynews.com/2020/03/25/coronavirus-bill-gates-predicted-pandemic-in-2015/.

22. Edwards M. The role and limitations of philanthropy. The Bellagio Initiative: the future of philanthropy and development in the pursuit of human wellbeing. Brighton: Institute of Development Studies; 2011.

Chapter 14. Pharmaceuticals and Other Global Health Topics

1. Miller LH, Rojas-Jaimes J, Low LM, Corbellini G. What historical records teach us about the discovery of quinine. Am J Trop Med Hyg. 2022. tpmd220404-tpmd.

2. World Health Organization. World Health Organization model list of essential medicines, 21st list, 2019. Geneva: WHO, 2019.

3. Webb JLA. Humanity's burden: a global history of malaria. Cambridge: Cambridge University Press; 2009.

4. Cueva-Agila A, Vélez-Mora D, Arias D, Curto M, Meimberg H, Brinegar C. Genetic characterization of fragmented populations of *Cinchona officinalis* L. (Rubiaceae), a threatened tree of the northern Andean cloud forests. Tree Genetics & Genomes. 2019;15(6):81. https://doi.org/10.1007/s11295-019-1393-y.

5. Crawford MJ. The Andean wonder drug: cinchona bark and imperial science in the Spanish Atlantic, 1630–1800. Pittsburgh, PA: University of Pittsburgh Press; 2016.

6. Harrison N. In celebration of the Jesuit's powder: a history of malaria treatment. The Lancet Infect Dis. 2015;15(10):1143. https://doi.org/10.1016/S1473-3099(15)00246-7.

7. Arnold D. Warm climates and western medicine: the emergence of tropical medicine, 1500–1900. Leiden (NL): BRILL; 2020.

8. Alchon SA. A pest in the land: New World epidemics in a global perspective. Albuquerque: University of New Mexico Press; 2003.

9. British Broadcasting Corporation. How Chinese traditional medicine helped beat malaria 2019. Available from: https://www.bbc.com/news/av/stories-47531213.

10. Faurant C. From bark to weed: the history of artemisinin. Parasite. 2011 Aug;18(3):215–18.

11. Weiyuan C. Ancient Chinese anti-fever cure becomes panacea for malaria. Bull World Health Organ. 2009;87(10):743.

12. Hsu E, Obringer F. *Qing hao* (Herba *Artemisiae annuae*) in the Chinese materia medica. Plants, health and healing: on the interface of ethnobotany and medical anthropology. In: Harris S, Hsu E, editors. Plants, health and healing: on the interface of ethnobotany and medical anthropology. New York: Oxford; 2010:83–130.

13. Centers for Disease Control and Prevention. Antibiotic resistance threats in the United States, 2019. Available from: https://ndc.services.cdc.gov/wp-content/uploads/Antibiotic-Resistance-Threats-in-the-United-States-2019.pdf.

14. O'Neill J, Chairman. Tackling drug-resistant infections globally: final report and recommendations. Review on Antimicrobial Resistance. 2016 May. https://wellcomecollection.org/works/thvwsuba.

15. Ventola CL. The antibiotic resistance crisis: part 1: causes and threats. Pharmacy and Therapeutics. 2015;40(4):277.

16. Antibiotic resistance: Cleveland Clinic; 2021 [cited 2023]. Available from: https://my.clevelandclinic.org/health/articles/21655-antibiotic -resistance.

17. Clarke I, editor. Science Museum. 2019. [cited 2023]. Tuberculosis: a fashionable disease? Available from: https://blog.sciencemuseum .org.uk/tuberculosis-a-fashionable-disease/.

18. Keshavjee S, Farmer PE. Tuberculosis, drug resistance, and the history of modern medicine. N Engl J Med. 2012;367(10):931–36.

19. Herzog H. History of tuberculosis. Respiration. 1998;65(1):5.

20. Pham TDM, Ziora ZM, Blaskovich MAT. Quinolone antibiotics. Medchemcomm. 2019;10(10):1719–39. Epub 2019/12/06. https:// doi.org/10.1039/c9md00120d. PubMed PMID: 31803393; PMCID: PMC6836748.

21. Yassin MA, Samson K, Wandwalo E, Grzemska M, Gegia M, Nwa-neri N, Hansen P, Kunii O. Performance-based technical support for drug-resistant TB responses: lessons from the Green Light Commit-tee. Int J Tuberc Lung Dis. 2020;24(1):22–27. https://doi.org/10.5588 /ijtld.19.0376.

22. World Health Organization. WHO consolidated guidelines on tuber-culosis module 4: treatment - drug-resistant tuberculosis treatment, 2022 Update. 2022.

23. World Health Organization. WHO announces landmark changes in treatment of drug-resistant tuberculosis. 2022.

24. Centers for Disease Control and Prevention. 2019 Antibiotic Resis-tance Threats Report. 2024 Mar. 20. Available from: https://www.cdc .gov/antimicrobial-resistance/data-research/threats/?CDC_AAref_Val= https://www.cdc.gov/drugresistance/biggest-threats.html.

25. Bush LM, Perez MT. The anthrax attacks 10 years later. Ann Intern Med. 2012;1201256(1 Pt 1):41. https://doi.org/10.7326/0003-4819 -155-12-201112200-00373.

26. US Centers for Disease Control and Prevention. History of anthrax. 2020 Dec 14. https://www.cdc.gov/anthrax/basics/anthrax-history .html (page removed).

27. Blevins SM, Bronze MS. Robert Koch and the 'golden age' of bacteriology. Int J Infect Dis. 2010;14(9):e744–51. https://doi.org /10.1016/j.ijid.2009.12.003.

28. Goetz T. The remedy: Robert Koch, Arthur Conan Doyle, and the quest to cure tuberculosis. New York: Gotham Books; 2014.

29. Louis Pasteur, null Chamberland, and null Roux. Summary report of the experiments conducted at Pouilly-Le-Fort, near Melun,

on the anthrax vaccination, 1881. Yale J Biol Med. 2002;75(1): 59–62.

30. Koch R. On the anthrax inoculation (1882). In: Carter KC; translator. Essays of Robert Koch. Connecticut: Greenwood Press; 1987:100.

31. Turnbull PCB. Anthrax vaccines: past, present and future. Vaccine. 1991 Aug;9(8):533–39. https://doi.org/10.1016/0264-410X(91)90237-Z.

32. Morris K. US military face punishment for refusing anthrax vaccine. Lancet. 1999 Jan;353(9147):130. https://doi.org/10.1016/S0140-6736(05)76173-0.

33. *Doe v. Rumsfeld.* Civil Action No. 03–707 (EGS) (D.D.C. Apr. 6, 2005).

34. Trust for America's Health. Remembering 9/11 and anthrax: public health's vital role in national defense. https://www.tfah.org/report-details/remembering-9-11-and-anthrax-public-healths-vital-role-in-national-defense/.

35. McNeil DG, Jr. Fauci on what working for Trump was really like. The New York Times. 2021 Jan 24. sec. Health. https://www.nytimes.com/2021/01/24/health/fauci-trump-covid.html.

36. Dowden H, Munro J. Trends in clinical success rates and therapeutic focus. Nat Rev Drug Discov. 2019 May;18(7):495–96. https://doi.org/10.1038/d41573-019-00074-z.

37. Lim S. The process and costs of drug development (2022). FTLOScience 2018 Jun 28. Updated 2023 Feb 6. https://ftloscience.com/process-costs-drug-development/.

38. United States Government Accountability Office. (2017). Drug industry: profits, research and development spending, and merger and acquisition deals Report to congressional requesters GAO-18-40. https://www.gao.gov/assets/gao-18-40.pdf.

39. Sun H. (2004). The road to Doha and beyond: some reflections on the TRIPS Agreement and public health. Eur J Int Law. 2004 Feb;15(1):123–50. https://doi.org/10.1093/ejil/15.1.123.

40. Fathi M, Peiravian F, Yousefi N. (2021). Impact of the trade-related aspect of Intellectual Property Rights Agreement on Pharmaceutical Industry in developing countries: a scoping review. Iranian Journal of Pharmaceutical Research: IJPR. 2021;20(4):339–51. https://doi.org/10.22037/ijpr.2021.115264.15282.

41. Hoen E't, Berger J, Calmy A, Moon S. (2011). Driving a decade of change: HIV/AIDS, patents and access to medicines for all. J Int AIDS Soc. 2011 Mar 27;14(1). https://doi.org/10.1186/1758-2652-14-15.

42. World Trade Organization. Declaration on the TRIPS Agreement and public health (WT/MIN(01)/DEC/2; WTO Ministerial). The Organization; 2001. https://www.wto.org/english/thewto_e/minist_e/min01_e/mindecl_trips_e.htm.

43. Rosenberg T. H.I.V. drugs cost $75 in Africa, $39,000 in the U.S. Does it matter? The New York Times. 2018 Sep 18. https://www.nytimes.com/2018/09/18/opinion/pricing-hiv-drugs-america.html.

44. Harrison C. Patent battle lines drawn as sofosbuvir gains approval. Nat Rev Drug Discov. 2014;13(1):12. https://doi.org/10.1038/nrd4220.

45. Médecins Sans Frontières. Appeal lodged against decision to uphold Gilead's patent on hepatitis C drug [Press Release]. 2018 Dec 5. https://www.msf.org/appeal-lodged-against-decision-uphold-gilead%E2%80%99s-patent-hepatitis-c-drug.

46. van de Ven N, Fortunak J, Simmons B, Ford N, Cooke G S, Khoo S, Hill A. Minimum target prices for production of direct-acting antivirals and associated diagnostics to combat hepatitis C virus. Hepatology. 2015 Mar 25;61(4):1174–82. https://doi.org/10.1002/hep.27641.

47. I-MAK. (n.d.). I-MAK's U.S. cases on Sofosbuvir. https://www.i-mak.org/cases/us-cases-hepatitis-c/.

48. Boseley S. Hepatitis C drug delayed by NHS due to high cost. The Guardian. 2015 Jan 16; https://www.theguardian.com/society/2015/jan/16/sofosbuvir-hepatitis-c-drug-nhs.

49. I-MAK. Gilead denied patent for hepatitis C drug sofosbuvir in India. 2015 Jan 14. https://www.i-mak.org/2015/01/14/gilead-denied-patent-for-hepatitis-c-drug-sofosbuvir-in-india/.

50. Gilead Sciences. Gilead announces generic licensing agreements to increase access to hepatitis C treatments in developing countries [Press Release]. 2014 Sep 15. https://www.gilead.com/news-and-press/press-room/press-releases/2014/9/gilead-announces-generic-licensing-agreements-to-increase-access-to-hepatitis-c-treatments-in-developing-countries.

51. Natco Pharma launches generic hepatitis C drug in India. The Economic Times. 2017 May 8. https://economictimes.indiatimes.com/industry/healthcare/biotech/pharmaceuticals/natco-pharma-launches-generic-hepatitis-c-drug-in-india/articleshow/58573146.cms?from=mdr.

52. World Bank Open Data. (n.d.). In: World Bank Open Data. Retrieved 2023 Jun 1. https://data.worldbank.org.

53. Wan F. New travel horizons: hepatitis C tourism from China. China
Real Time Report. Wall Street Journal. 2016 Mar 30. https://web
.archive.org/web/20170322203726/http://blogs.wsj.com/chinare
altime/2016/03/30/new-travel-horizons-hepatitis-c-tourism-from
-china/.

Chapter 15. Promoting Positive Change

1. Rosenberg M, Foege WH. Nine lessons for the next generation.
[Interview with M Rosenberg and W Foege]. Contagious Conversa-
tions podcast. 2023 Feb. [Available from CDCfoundation.org].
2. Scheele LA. The Indianapolis Literary Club 2006–2007: 128th Year
Leonard A. Scheele: Hoosier Sage of Science and Public Health
Essayist: Stephen J. Jay M.D. Read on Monday, October 16, 2006,
at the regular meeting of the Indianapolis Literary Club, Park Tudor
School, Indianapolis, Indiana.

cervical cancer, 91, 260–61
Chamberlain, Joseph, 93
charity, 84, 151, 189, 192, 198, 207.
    See also philanthropy
Chernobyl incident, 10–11
child health programs, 74–78, 115,
    128, 212
Child Survival and Development
    Revolution, 145
China: aid by, 62, 120–25, 129; aid
    to, 72–74, 82, 120–21; and Gavi,
    211–12; and malaria, 62, 122, 239;
    One China policy, 123–24, 131–32;
    and TRIPS Agreement, 257
China International Development
    Cooperation Agency (CIDCA),
    120–25
China State Construction Engineering
    Corporation, 123
Chinese traditional medicine, 72, 122,
    239
Chlamydia trachomatis, 73, 231
chloroquine, 239
cholera: colonial approaches to,
    27–28, 47–48; and global health
    security, 65; and Haiti earthquake
    (2010), 103; and militaries, 47–48,
    65; reporting on in US, 86; trans-
    port and expansion of, 42–43; and
    water, 27–28, 47, 92, 103
Christian Health Association of
    Lesotho, 71
Christian Medical College Vellore, 76
Christian Medical Commission (CMC),
    80–82
Christian Missions in Many Lands
    (CMML), 40–41
Christmas seals, 152
chronic disease, 233, 262, 264
Churches Health Association of
    Zambia, 71
Churchill, Winston, x, 143
CIA (Central Intelligence Agency), 66,
    108–10
cinchona bark, 234–35, 237–38
Cipla, 254
Cleveland, Harlan, 271

climate change, 263
Clinton, Bill, 163, 252
clofazimine, 80
Clostridiodes difficiles, 245
Coalition for Epidemic Preparedness
    Innovations (CEPI), 141, 142
Cochrane, Robert Greenhill, 79–80
Cold War, 59–60, 105–6, 155–56,
    208
College, Thomas, 74
colonialism: and bilateral programs,
    104; and cholera, 27–28, 47–48;
    and competition in global health,
    30–34; and disease dynamics, 21–25;
    and famine, 36; and germ theory,
    29–30; and Indigenous mortality,
    22–23; influence on modern global
    health, 45–46; and leprosy, 78–79;
    and malaria, 22, 23–24, 25, 26,
    36–37, 44–45, 234–37; and medical
    missionary approach, 67–70, 82;
    and militaries, 25, 27–28, 47–48,
    51; and multilateral organizations,
    41–45; negative impact on global
    health, x, 4, 35–37, 46; and plague,
    22, 47–48; and power of local inter-
    mediaries, 37–41; and slavery, 23–24;
    and sleeping sickness, 30–34, 36;
    and traditional medicine, 40–41,
    236–37; and United Nations, 41, 43;
    and White mortality, 24–28, 51, 54;
    and WHO, 41, 43–45; and yellow
    fever, 22, 23, 25, 26, 52–53, 54
Commission for Technical Coopera-
    tion in Africa South of the Sahara
    (CCTA), 44
Communicable Disease Center, 58
community health workers: *accom-
    pagnateurs* model, 169–71; and
    BRAC, 174; and Chinese medical
    aid, 121–22; and Global Fund,
    137; and NGOs, 174; and PIH,
    133, 169–71; salaries, 169, 170;
    and WHO, 129, 133. *See also*
    healthcare workers
Company of Merchants Trading to
    Africa, 26

education: and Becoming Better
  Ancestors, 269–71; Black medical
  schools, 98, 101; early academic
  programs, 83–102; and Flexner
  Report, 85, 97–98, 101; future of,
  263–66; and hands-on experience,
  101, 265, 266; of women and
  GOBI-FF, 145; of women physicians, 76
Ehanire, Osagie, 125
Eliot, Charles W., 89
End Fund, 230
English Royal African Company, 26
Enterobacterales, Carbapenem-
  resistant, 245
Epidemic Intelligence Service (EIS),
  60–61
epidemics and pandemics: cholera, 42,
  47–48; and colonialism, 27, 36–37;
  Ebola, 64; and Gates, 213; H1N1,
  64; H5N1, 127; influenza, 84, 93;
  likeliness of future, 4; malaria,
  36–37; and NGOs, 179–81; plague,
  47–48; preparedness training, 62;
  sleeping sickness, 31, 36; surveillance, 60–61
Exotic Pathology Society, 52
Expanded Program on Immunization,
  186

faith groups, 17–18, 151, 161–62.
  See also religious missions
family planning, 115, 135, 145, 212,
  262–63
famine, 15, 36, 158
Farmer, Paul, 133, 167–68, 171, 244
Fauci, Anthony, 252
FBI, 246, 258
female genital mutilation, 116, 167
Feminist International Assistance
  Policy, 115–16
Finlay, Carlos, 53
Flexner, Abraham, 85, 87, 88–89, 97,
  99, 101
Flexner Report, 85, 97–98, 101
food aid and security, 104, 145, 148,
  152–54, 164, 175, 194

Food and Agriculture Organization of
  the UN, 65, 221
Food and Drug Administration (FDA),
  140
Ford Foundation, 207
Foster, Stan, 13
Foundation for Innovative New
  Diagnostics (FIND), 141
France: and Biafran War, 157; and
  colonialism, 24–25, 26, 31, 32–33,
  34–35, 36, 51–52, 54; and resis-
  tance to multilateral organizations,
  43–45; and tropical medicine, 50;
  and tuberculosis, 199; and World
  Bank funding, 133
Frost, Wade Hampton, 90

G8, 115, 135
G20 Summit, 211
Gap, 139
Garcilaso de la Vega, 237
Gates, Bill, 134, 206, 210–11, 213,
  216
Gates, Bill, Sr., 206
Gates, Frederick T., 84, 192, 193, 195,
  196
Gates, Melinda, 206, 212, 216
Gates Foundation. *See* Bill & Melinda
  Gates Foundation
Gavi (Global Alliance for Vaccines
  and Immunization), 187, 209–12,
  258
Gayle, Helene, 166
gender equity, 115–16, 165–66
General Education Board (GEB), 195
generics, 253, 254, 255
Geneva Convention, 63, 151, 250
Germany: Berlin Blockade, 154; and
  bioweapons, 250; and CARE, 165;
  and colonialism, 31, 32, 33; and
  pharmaceutical industry, 30; and
  rivalries in global health, 51
germ theory, 29–34, 204, 248–50
Ghebreyesus, Tedros Adhanom,
  127–28, 141–42
Gilead, 257
Giving Pledge, 213

GlaxoSmithKline, 230
Global Affairs Canada, 114–17
Global AIDS Act, 111
Global Alliance for Vaccines and
    Immunization (Gavi), 187, 209–12,
    258
Global Fund for AIDS, Tuberculosis,
    and Malaria, 111, 112, 114, 135–40,
    255
global health: career considerations,
    260, 261–63; future of, 260–71;
    mentorship, 265–66; philosophy,
    265–66
Global Health Security Agenda (GHSA),
    64–65
Global Malaria Eradication Program,
    203
Global Programme on AIDS, 160
Global Public Private Partnership, 210
GOBI (Growth charts, Oral rehydra-
    tion, Breastfeeding, and Immuniza-
    tion), 144–46, 208
GOBI-FF, 145–46
Goebbels, Joseph, 143
Goldsmith, Grace A., 100
gonorrhea, 245
Gorgas, William, 53–54, 55–56,
    200–201
Gowan, Yakubu, 13
Graham, Wendy, 97
Grandmaison, Olivier Le Cour, 34–35,
    51
Grant, Jim, 144–45, 146, 185–86, 187
Grassi, Giovanni, 53
Greene, Jerome, 87, 88, 89
guaiac, 236
Guinea worm eradication, 11–12,
    13–14, 260, 263

H1N1 (swine flu), 64
H5N1 (bird flu), 127
Haiti: colonialism in, 21–25; earth-
    quake (2010), 62, 103, 171, 182;
    and PIH, 167–69
Hansen, Gerhard Armauer, 79
Hansen's disease. See leprosy
Harper, Stephen, 115

Harvard University, 50, 87–88, 89,
    213
Hatfill, Steven, 246
Hay–Bunau-Varilla Treaty, 545
healthcare workers: "barefoot doc-
    tors," 121–22, 129, 239; and Global
    Fund, 137–38; medical personnel
    programs from Cuba, 117–19; as
    military targets, 63; and NGOs,
    156–58; and Orbis International,
    176; salaries, 113, 118, 138, 169,
    170; suspicion of, 66, 110. See also
    community health workers
Health Emergencies Programme, 131
health inequities, 129, 130, 133–34,
    262, 270–71
heartworm, 219, 220
Heiser, Victor, 95
hepatitis, 109–10, 188, 231, 256–57,
    261
Hepburn, Audrey, 148
Hernández, Francisco, 237
Hill, Bradford, 96
Hill, J. Lister, 7
Hilton, Conrad, 215
Hilton Foundation Board, 215
Hippocrates, 27, 241
HIV/AIDS: and bilateral programs,
    105, 110–14; and Carter Center,
    13; Doha Declaration, 163–64, 255;
    and Gates Foundation, 213, 215;
    and multilateral programs, 135–40;
    and NGOs, 158–64, 170; PEPFAR
    program, 110–14, 139, 255; pro-
    tests, 148, 162; (RED) campaign,
    139–40; treatment, 162–64, 213,
    254–56; and tuberculosis, 244; and
    United Nations, 111, 161; vaccine,
    62, 215; and WHO, 160, 161
hookworm: and Flexner, 101; and
    Leiper, 93; and pharmaceutical
    philanthropy, 230; reduction in,
    261; and Rockefeller Foundation,
    56, 84, 88, 93, 195–99
Hoover, Herbert, 153
Hopkins, Don, 11, 12
horizontal programs, 168, 208

public health, 27–28, 47–48; competition in global health, 51–52; and disaster relief, 62; disease control approaches, 47–48; and Geneva Convention, 63, 151; and global health security, 64–65; and malaria, 57–59, 235, 238–39; mortality from disease, 24–28, 51; naval origins of global health, 49–51; and NGOs, 153; and plague, 47–48; positive impact on global health, x, 4, 62, 66; and quinine, 235, 238–39; tensions between goals, 61–66; and tropical medicine, 92–93; and USAID, 108–9; and World Bank, 134–35; and yellow fever, 52–54, 58, 65

milk, 194

Millennium Development Goals, 211

missionaries. *See* religious missions

Mission to Lepers, 79

Mond, Alfred, 96

Mond Committee, 95–96

monkeypox, 3

Moores, John, 14, 227

Morbidity and Mortality Weekly Report, 86

Morgan, Isabel, 90

Morrison, Robert, 72

mortality: CDC morbidity and mortality reports, 86; and colonialism, 22–29, 51–54, 57; infant mortality and slavery, 29; maternal mortality, 97; military mortality from disease, 24–28, 51; preventable deaths, 6, 7, 10

mosquitoes, 23–24, 53–57, 58, 200, 201–3, 228

Mountin, Joseph Walter, 58

multilateral programs, 127–47; and ACT-Accelerator, 140–42; vs. bilateral, 103–4, 112, 147; challenges of, 146; and colonialism, 41–45; defined, 103–4; and Global Affairs Canada, 114; Global Fund, 135–40; and hybrid organizations, 185–88; UNICEF, 142–46; WHO, 127–32, 147; World Bank, 132–35, 146–47

Museveni, Yoweri, 13

Muslim Solidarity Trust Fund, 71

Mycobacterium leprae, 79

Mycobacterium tuberculosis, 242

Nakajima, Hiroshi, 147

Nansen, Fridtjof, 154

Nansen Refugee Award, 177

Napoleon I, 24, 25

National Association for the Study and Prevention of Tuberculosis, 152

National Defense Malaria Control Activities, 57–58

National Institutes of Health, 3, 50, 209, 213

National Security Resources Board, 60

naval origins of global health, 49–51

needles, bifurcated, 224

neglected diseases, 11–13, 212

Netherlands and colonialism, 30, 236, 238

NGOs (nongovernmental organizations), 148–84; challenges of, 181–84; and crises and disasters, 164, 176, 179–81, 184; defined, 149; development post-WWII, 152–58; and faith groups, 151, 161–62; and food aid, 152–54; funding, 149, 155–56, 157, 182, 183; and Global Affairs Canada, 115; golden era (1990s), 158–76; and HIV/AIDS, 158–64, 170; and hybrid organizations, 185–88; increase in, 149; and militaries, 153; and modern-day partnerships, 176–81; origins of, 150–52; and pandemics, 179–81; and refugees, 148, 154, 176–79; role of today, 181–83; and salaries, 166, 169, 170, 182; as term, 150; and tuberculosis, 151–52, 168–69; types of, 149–50

NGO Watch, 182

Nigeria: aid to, 11–12, 13, 14, 123, 125, 211; and Doctors Without Borders origins, 156–57

night blindness, 89–90

9Lessons.org, 267–69

Thoburn, Isabella, 75
Thomas, D. W., 75
Thorpe, Jim, 13
tobacco, 7, 18, 96, 130
Tocqueville, Alexis de, 150
Touré, Amadou Toumani, 13
trachoma, 12–13, 14, 73, 188,
    231–32, 261
traditional medicine, 40–41, 72, 122,
    234–40
TRIPS Agreement (Trade-Related
    Aspects of Intellectual Property
    Rights), 163–64, 253–57
tropical medicine programs, 30,
    49–50, 62, 91–100, 101
Trudeau, Justin, 115–16
Truman, Harry S., 106
Trump, Donald, 2, 104, 116, 128,
    131, 139
Trypanosoma brucei spp., 31
tsetse fly, 31–32
Tu, Youyou, 122
tuberculosis, 29, 101, 151–52,
    168–69, 199, 240–45
Tulane School of Hygiene and
    Tropical Medicine, 97–100, 101
typhus, 22

UNICEF: and ACT-Accelerator, 141;
    and Gavi, 209–10; and hybrid orga-
    nizations, 185–87; and malaria, 44;
    as multilateral program, 142–46;
    and primary healthcare, 129; and
    vertical approach, 208; and vita-
    mins, 90
Unitaid, 141
United Kingdom: and Biafran War,
    157; and bioweapons, 250–51;
    and colonialism, 25–28, 37–41, 44,
    51; and quinine, 238; and tropical
    medicine, 49
United Nations: and colonialism, 41,
    43; and Global Fund, 135; and
    Global Health Security Agenda,
    65; and HIV/AIDS, 111, 161; and
    hybrid organizations, 186–87;
    and malaria, 44; and NGOs, 150;

origins of, 41; and refugees, 154,
    176–79; and river blindness, 221;
    and sustainability, 130, 166; and
    Task Force for Child Survival, 9
United Nations Development Pro-
    gramme (UNDP), 9, 186–87, 221
United Nations High Commissioner
    for Refugees (UNHCR), 154,
    176–79
United Nations Relief and Rehabilita-
    tion Administration (UNRRA), 128,
    143–44
United States: and bilateral programs,
    104–14; and bioweapons, 251;
    influence on Global Fund, 138–39;
    influence on World Bank, 135; life
    expectancy in, 17–18; and WHO
    support, 2, 128, 131
United States Leadership Against HIV/
    AIDS, Tuberculosis, and Malaria
    Act, 111
United States Public Health Service
    (USPHS), 50, 51, 86, 193
USAID (US Agency for International
    Development): as bilateral program,
    106–10; and Cuban medical assis-
    tance, 118; founding, 106–7; and
    HIV/AIDS, 213; and hybrid organi-
    zations, 186–87; and NGOs, 155,
    156; and PEPFAR, 111; and polio,
    109; and river blindness, 187, 220;
    and smallpox, 105
USAMRIID (US Army's Medical
    Research Institute of Infectious
    Diseases), 246

vaccines: anthrax, 249–50, 252; and
    Carter Center, 12; COVID-19, 3,
    141–42, 258, 264; development, 30,
    62, 209, 261; Ebola, 62; and Gates
    Foundation, 209, 211; and Gavi,
    187, 209–12, 258; hepatitis, 109–10,
    231, 261; hesitancy, x, 109–10, 211,
    261, 264; HIV, 62, 215; HPV, 91,
    261; and life expectancy, 18; ma-
    laria, 62; pneumonia, 195; polio,
    90, 109, 211; and reduction in

vaccines (*cont.*)
cancers, 91, 231, 260–61; ring vaccination, ix–x; smallpox, ix–x, 129–30, 193; tuberculosis, 242; yellow fever, 195, 201. *See also* immunization, child
Vagelos, Roy, 219, 220, 221, 223
Vasa, 266–67
Vasal, Surinder, 16
vertical programs, 121, 168, 208
Village Loans and Savings Associations, 166
Village Organizations, 173
Villegas, Evangelina, 16
Vincent, George Edgar, 96, 202
vitamins, 89–90

Waksman, Selman, 242
War Relief Control Board (US), 153
Warren, A. J., 201
Warren, Ken, 185
Watson, Bill, 7
Welch, William H., 88–89
Welch-Rose Report, 86
Wellcome Trust, 141, 216
Wellman, Frederick Creighton, 98–100
Wheat Ridge Foundation, 214
whipworms, 223, 230
White, Thomas J., 168
WHO (World Health Organization): and ACT-Accelerator, 141; and Canadian aid, 114; and child immunization, 186–87; and colonialism, 41, 43–45; and community health workers, 129, 133; and COVID-19, 2, 127–28, 132, 140; and Declaration of Alma-Ata, 129, 179, 208; and faith groups, 82; funding, 128, 130–31, 132, 208, 210; and Gavi, 209–10, 258; and Global Health Security Agenda, 65; and HIV/AIDS, 160, 161; and hybrid organizations, 185–87; and IHC, 203, 207; and lymphatic filariasis, 229–30; and malaria, 44–45, 203–4; morbidity and mortality reporting, 128; as

multilateral program, 127–32, 147; origins of, 41; and river blindness, 187, 220, 221, 222, 227; and Rockefeller Foundation, 207, 215; and smallpox, x, 83, 129–30; and Task Force for Child Survival, 9; and tobacco, 130; and tuberculosis, 243–45; US exit from, 2, 128
Williams, Cicely, 16–17
women: and BRAC, 172–74; and CARE, 165–67; female education, 145; female genital mutilation, 116, 167; and Gates Foundation, 212; and gender equity, 115–16, 165–66; and Global Affairs Canada, 115–16; and HIV/AIDS programs, 161; as medical missionaries, 74–78; and medical missions in India, 74–78, 82; and NGOs, 172–74
Women's Union Missionary Society of America for Heathen Lands, 75
Woodworth, John, 50–51
World Bank: and ACT-Accelerator, 141; and colonialism, 41; DALYs, 19, 134, 146, 216, 243; and hybrid organizations, 186–87; as multilateral program, 132–35, 146–47; and NGOs, 155; origins of, 41, 133; and river blindness, 135, 221, 223, 226, 227; and Task Force for Child Survival, 9; and tuberculosis, 243; US influence on, 135
World Council of Churches, 80
World Food Programme, 175
World Organization for Animal Health, 65
World Trade Organization, 163, 253–57
World Vision, 178, 182
worm infections: Guinea worm, 11–12, 13–14, 260, 263; and hybrid organizations, 188; ivermectin for, 223; and pharmaceutical philanthropy, 228–31; roundworms, 223, 230, 261; whipworms, 223, 230. *See also* hookworm; lymphatic filariasis

Wuchereria, 228
Wyeth Pharmaceuticals, 224
Wyman, Walter, 99

xerophthalmia (night blindness),
   89–90
X-rays, 242

yellow fever: and colonialism, 22,
   23, 25, 26, 52–53, 54; and global
health security, 65; and IHC, 199;
and militaries, 52–54, 58, 65; and
mosquitoes, 23–24, 53–57; national
reporting in US, 86; and Panama
Canal Zone, 54–57, 200; and race,
56–57; and Rockefeller Foundation,
195, 199, 200–201; and slavery,
23–24, 28–29; vaccines, 195, 201

Zemurray, Samuel, 99

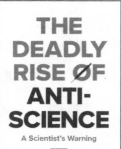
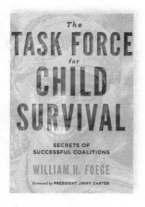
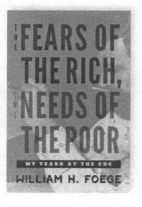